FOR MY FAMILY.
YOU ARE EVERYTHING.

How to Eat Paleo
(When You Don't Live in a Cave)

The information in this book is not intended as a substitute for medical
advice. Consult your physician or nutrition expert for information
regarding any type of nutrition or medical plan.

ISBN 978-0-9968434-1-6
Library of Congress Control Number 2016909597
Printed in the United States
Paperback, First Printing July 2016
Book design, Jesse Groves

Smiling Water Group
P.O. Box 50818
Santa Barbara, CA 93150

www.smilingwatergroup.com

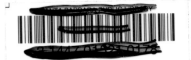

How to Eat Paleo

(When You Don't Live in a Cave)

CYNTHIA SPIVEY

ILLUSTRATED BY JOYA ROSE GROVES

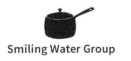

Smiling Water Group

CONTENTS

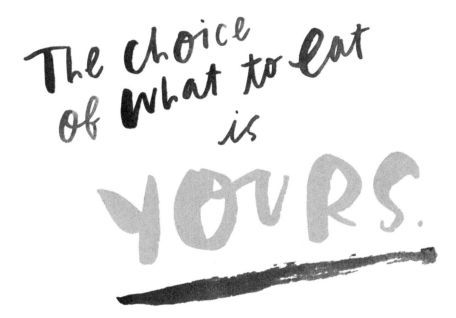

The choice of what to eat is YOURS.

INTRODUCTION

When I started eating Paleo, it was difficult to explain the concept to my friends, most of whom had never heard of the unusual and seemingly very limited "diet." Paleo was brushed off as a crazy fad that I would soon get over and then return to normal.

About six months later, when it became noticeable that I had lost weight and was looking better than I had in over ten years, people were surprised I was still eating Paleo. "How much longer are you going to do this?" was the common question I was asked as I once again declined a piece of bread at lunch or dinner. The most entertaining part was the look of confusion and complete disbelief when I explained that I was not "doing" anything. This was my new normal. I was going to eat primarily Paleo forever.

After about nine months, some of those same people wanted to understand more about what I was doing and how to do it. And in the year following that, almost everyone who spent any time with me, and especially those who ate dinner at my house, commented that they might actually be able to embrace eating this way. More questions were asked, many of which were easy to answer, while some were a bit harder for me since science is not my passion. But they were the same questions I asked myself when I started researching the Paleo way of eating.

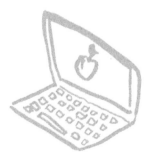

One common question was "What book would you recommend to learn about Paleo?" There are excellent websites and books for recipes and scientific information, but I hadn't yet found a concise, easy-to-understand guide to get someone started and inspire them to try eating Paleo. I believe that is because Paleo did not originate as a commercial diet. No one owns the idea of Paleo eating, so there is no official guidebook. Paleo has developed over decades with the leadership of a few Paleo gurus, plus many others that are newer to the Paleo scene (see the Resources page for a current selection of Paleo experts) who contribute excellent information on the lifestyle and science of eating Paleo.

My knowledge was gained by hundreds of hours of reading and research, using a vast array of sources from out-of-print food history books to current websites. I discovered that there are many variables to eating Paleo and the choice of what to eat is yours. No one will tell you exactly what to do, which is why people sometimes find it confusing. Paleo is a "diet" that requires some education and experimentation. There are some yeses, some noes, and a whole lot of maybes.

For my own sanity, I started compiling the information, interpreting it to fit today's lifestyle. We don't live in caves, nor do we hunt and gather our own food, so Paleo is an interpretation of a paleolithic lifestyle that no longer exists. It makes sense that there are many variables.

My personal research resulted in this guidebook, which I hope helps you navigate those variables and find a Paleo lifestyle that works for you.

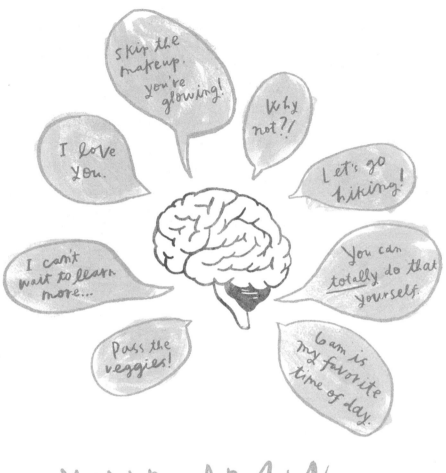

YOUR BRAIN on PALEO

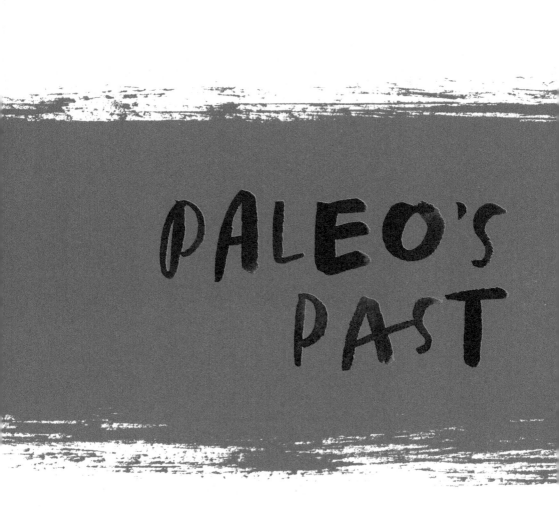

SOME INVENTIONS of CIVILIZATION have caused more HARM than GOOD.

WONDER

The evolution of man as a thinking human being has been traced to the introduction of meat, specifically cooked meat. While this is just one theory of evolution, the evidence points to this idea that eating digestible, nutrient-dense animal protein was a catalyst for the evolution of an advanced society. When man began eating cooked meat, the size of the gut decreased and the size of the brain increased, fostering the belief that protein is "brain food."

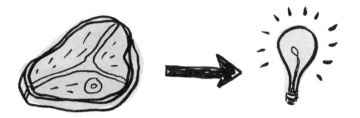

Four million years ago, a type of ape-man lived in trees. When the food sources in trees became scarce, the ape-man came down and began foraging small animals such as lizards, tortoises, squirrels and insects. This developed into hurling rocks at larger animals, which required the ape-man to eventually move on two legs. The forelegs adapted into hands with dexterity to create tools.

By a half million years ago, the ape-man had evolved to a man-ape or Homo erectus, which could hunt large game like buffalo, venison and boar. The man-ape had fire but had not yet begun cooking, resulting in a short life span due to vitamin deficiencies, malnutrition, plant poisoning and contaminated food.

Once cooking emerged, indigestible nutrition became digestible. Heat breaks down fibers and releases proteins and carbohydrates in food, increasing the nutritive value. Between 200,000 BC and 40,000 BC, larger-brained Homo sapiens and Neanderthals emerged. They were skilled hunters and fishermen who were developing refined tools and knowledge of food preservation.

From about 10,000 BC to 3,000 BC Homo sapiens boomed and civilization was born. They created villages and towns, discovered farming and created medicinal potions. The workload was spread among the village, and mankind thrived. This growth of civilization, culture and invention has continued into our current day.

However, some inventions of civilization have caused us more harm than good. Commonly available grains are no longer full of nutrients. Meat and

PALEO

is an attempt to give our bodies the chance to function

OPTIMALLY

in a world where much of our food is

NOT OPTIMAL.

dairy from cows that are fed grain and filled with antibiotics are not good for optimal health, neither for us nor the animals. It is only in the past decade or two, through the voices of whole food advocates, that we are beginning to understand the negative effects that innovation in techniques and processes of agriculture—including the use of pesticides—can have on our food. These foods are no longer the nutrient-dense foods of our ancestors.

The concept of Paleo is an attempt to allow our bodies to function optimally in a world where much of our food is not optimal. Eating Paleo returns our nutrition to the level of early Homo sapiens and Neanderthals, when food was freshly harvested and extremely dense in nutrients.

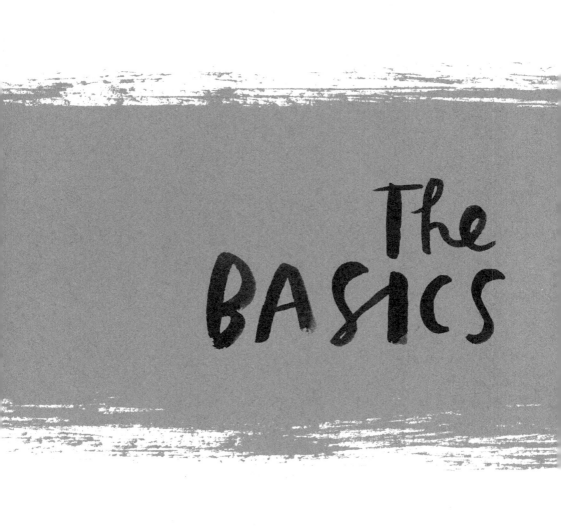

The
BASICS

DIY PALEO KIT

EASY!

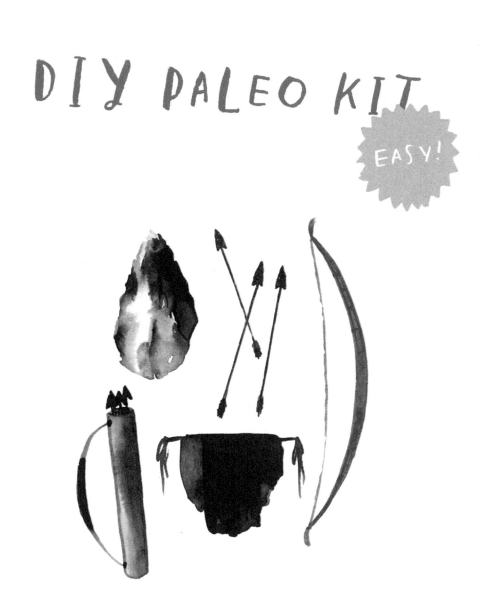

What Is Paleo?

Paleo is a choice to eat real food (with no calorie counting), focusing on eating: plenty of vegetables; well-sourced meat, fish and poultry; nuts and seeds; and fruit; with minimal starch, sugar and dairy.

Paleo eating is based on the nutritional characteristics of what Paleolithic man ate, choosing the most nutrient-dense foods available today. In Paleolithic times, foods varied by location and the sources that were available. Variables exist when eating a modern Paleo diet as well. Eat what works for you within the guidelines.

So... I can only eat what CAVEMEN ate?

Paleo is based on the diet of cavemen, not trying to replicate what was eaten 10,000 years ago. The idea is to eat unprocessed, whole foods that are rich in nutrients ("nutrient-dense") and avoid eating foods that can contribute to poor health, such as foods that contain calories but few nutrients.

What is nutrient-dense food?

Nutrients per calorie determine the nutrient density of a food. Lean meat has high nutrient density. Donuts have negative nutrient density.

WHY eat Paleo?

You will feel great, look great and your sharpened mind will challenge you to achieve new levels of purpose in your life.

Many Paleo enthusiasts have professed relief from symptoms of a variety of health issues, including a host of autoimmune-related diseases like inflammatory bowel, rheumatoid arthritis, type 1 diabetes, and multiple sclerosis.

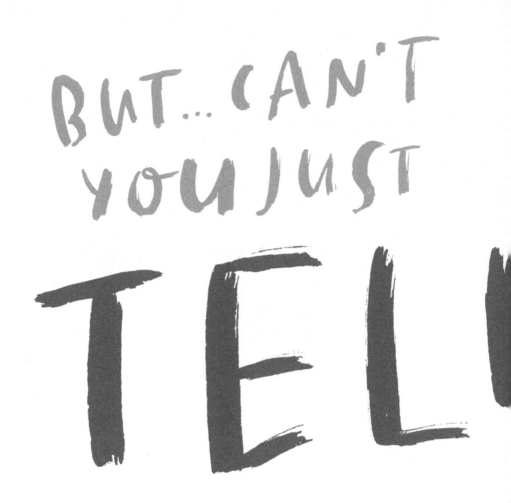

BUT... CAN'T YOU JUST TELL

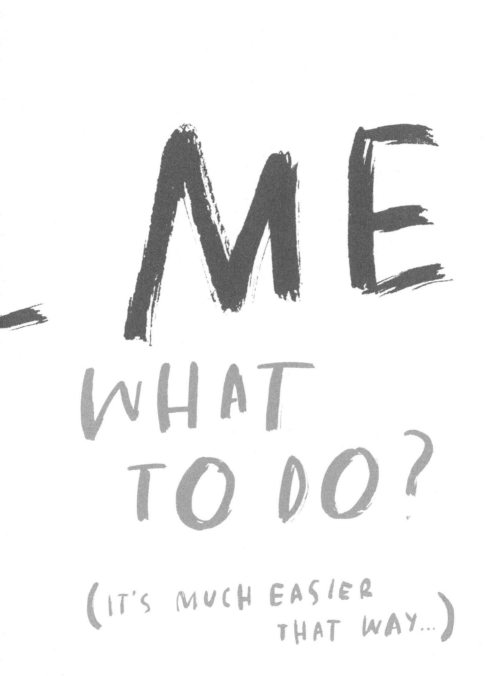

– ME
WHAT
TO DO?

(IT'S MUCH EASIER
THAT WAY...)

17

How does Paleo work?

Eating protein at every meal, with nutrient-dense fat and carbohydrates, helps your blood sugar levels remain consistent, reducing the peaks and dives of energy that make it difficult to function at your optimal level. Animal protein provides your brain with the nutrients it needs to function optimally. Eliminating grains and legumes reduces inflammation in your body caused by anti-nutrients present in those foods. Eating nutrient-dense foods and limiting sugar allows you to eat the amount your body needs to perform and reduces cravings for empty calories.

How do I get started?

Buying this book is a great start! You get to decide how to proceed from here. Some people dive right in for the first thirty days (which is recommended to identify any allergies or intolerances), easing up after their body is cleansed and they are free of old habits and unhealthy cravings. Others prefer to take it slow and wade in, one step at a time.

Can't you just TELL ME what to do?

Paleo isn't one-size-fits-all. You get to choose what you eat (within the Paleo framework), how much you eat and when you eat it! This guide will answer your questions and give you a place to start. Once you learn the basics, Paleo is amazingly simple to follow because there is no calorie counting, and you get to eat the foods you like on the schedule you choose.

RIGHT WAYS to LIVE PALEO

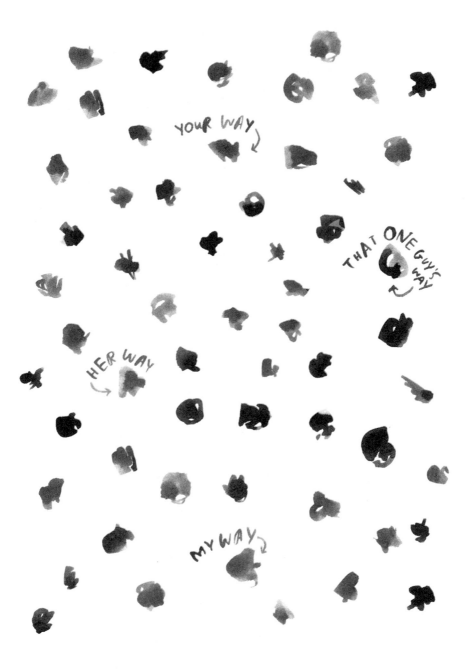

The PALEO TABLE

(WHAT to EAT)

What "table", you ask?
IT CAN BE ANY
TABLE, REALLY

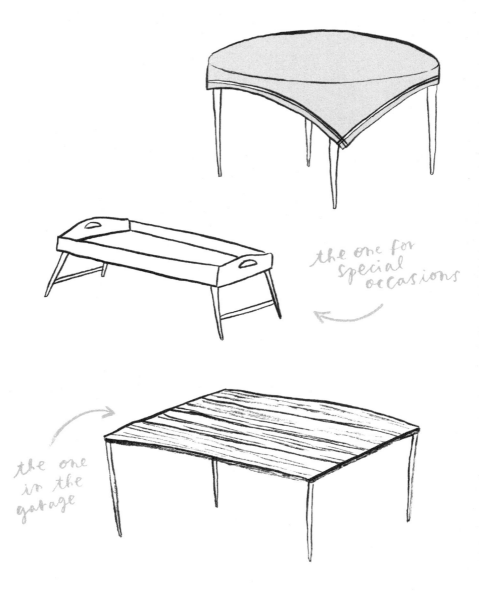

the one for special occasions

the one in the garage

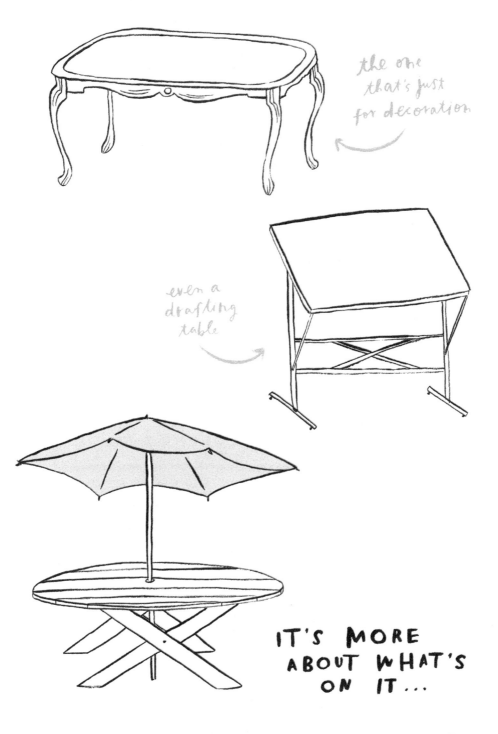

the one
that's just
for decoration

even a
drafting
table

IT'S MORE
ABOUT WHAT'S
ON IT...

What's ON the Paleo Table

EAT or DRINK LOTS

VEGETABLES

ANIMAL PROTEIN
meat, fish, eggs

ORGAN MEATS
(offal)

BONE MARROW
& BROTH

WATER

EAT or DRINK SOME

FRUIT & BERRIES

AVOCADO

FERMENTED
PLANT FOODS

SWEET POTATOES

FRESH GREEN
LEGUMES
*green beans,
snow peas,
sugar snap peas*

COFFEE & TEA

EAT or DRINK LITTLE

BACON

NUTS & SEEDS

DARK CHOCOLATE

DRIED FRUIT

WHITE RICE,
QUINOA,
SPROUTED LEGUMES

WHITE POTATOES

DAIRY
milk, cheese, yogurt

VEGETABLE JUICE,
SMOOTHIES,
KOMBUCHA

ALCOHOL

USE for COOKING & FLAVOR

HONEY, MAPLE SYRUP as sweeteners

BUTTER, GHEE, COCONUT OIL, OLIVE OIL

ANIMAL FATS lard, duck fat

COLD-PRESSED AVOCADO or NUT OILS

VINEGAR, FRUIT JUICE

NUT & COCONUT FLOURS

WHAT'S OFF the PALEO TABLE

GRAINS including corn

GLUTEN found in many grains

LEGUMES exceptions noted

SOY

PROCESSED FOODS

REFINED SUGAR

REFINED OILS

BEVERAGES CONTAINING SUGAR, CHEMICALS, or MADE FROM GRAINS

Why is it ON or OFF the Table?

Eat or Drink Lots

Vegetables can be eaten in large quantity, as many as you want, in lots of different colors. Vegetables provide the base alkaline to balance the acid in your body. Potatoes and sweet potatoes are limited.

Animal Protein should be eaten every day and preferably at every meal. Good choices are eggs, meats, poultry, fish and seafood. Try to get the best quality, freshest products you can find. Grass-fed and pasture-raised products are top of the list. Spam does not make the list.

Eggs are a wonderful source of protein and nutrients as long as you eat the whole egg. The most beneficial nutrients in eggs, including choline, which is helpful to the liver and memory, are found in the yolk. Eat the entire egg! Egg white omelets are just silly.

Organ Meats (Offal) are good for you. Organ meats (liver, heart, etc.) and other non-muscle parts (feet, tongue, etc.) are some of the most nutrient-dense foods available. Won't your mother be proud when you request liver and onions for dinner?

Bone Marrow and Bone Broth contain many nutrients, including minerals and amino acids that are difficult to get from other foods.

Water is the best thing to drink. Hydrate often.

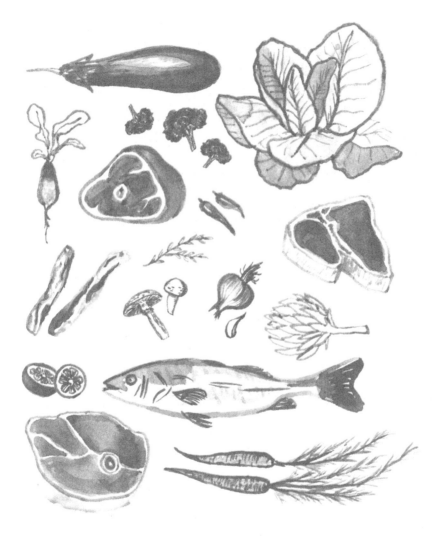

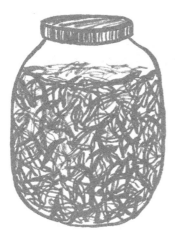

SOUR
KRAUT

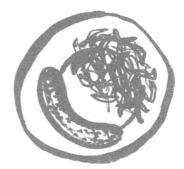

SWEET
DINNER

Eat or Drink Some

Fruit and Berries of all colors and all varieties are good, but try to eat your protein and veggies first because fruit has high sugar content. Monitor total intake of fruit if you have weight or insulin problems. The best fruits are berries. Less favorable fruits are bananas and pineapple due to higher sugar content.

Avocado is a fruit that is low in sugar, full of good fat and so simple to serve that it deserves a separate mention.

Fermented Plant Foods like sauerkraut and pickles are beneficial to your gut health. They contain good bacteria, also known as probiotics, and enzymes that keep your gut happy. Be aware that fermented foods are typically very salty.

Sweet Potatoes are a high-carb, starchy vegetable that can be consumed in limited portions. They are high in fiber and nutrients—and are void of some anti-nutrients like saponins and lectins—but they do contain oxalates, which are anti-nutrients that can prevent mineral absorption.

Fresh Green Legumes with edible pods like green beans, snow peas and sugar snap peas can be eaten in moderation. Legumes are typically a no-no because of anti-nutrients (phytic acid, which binds to nutrients preventing absorption, and lectins, which damage the intestinal wall.) However, the greener they are, the less anti-nutrients the legumes contain.

Coffee and Tea are okay in reasonable amounts. Reasonable is what works for you. If you feel jittery, have acid reflux or are not sleeping well, try cutting back on tea or coffee.

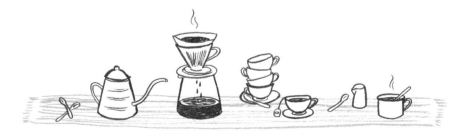

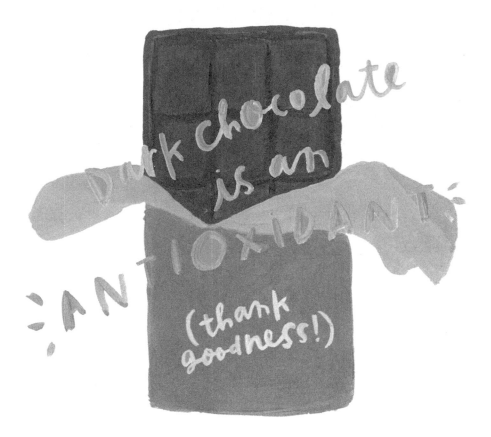

Dark chocolate is an ANTIOXIDANT (thank goodness!)

Eat or Drink Little

Bacon must be well sourced. The best bacon is from pasture-raised pigs and contains no added ingredients except salt and spices. Because so much bacon does not reach all these standards, it should be consumed in small quantities. If you have a reliable source, you can up the intake.

Nuts and Seeds are high in protein, and you can eat all types but consider them a snack or condiment, not a main course, because they are high in calories and contain small amounts of anti-nutrients. They do make an excellent food for travel. Some Paleo experts do not recommend chia seeds because they believe the anti-nutrients outweigh the benefits and the gel-like coating may impair digestion. It is important to note that peanuts are legumes, not nuts.

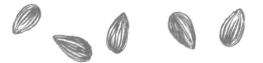

Dark Chocolate and Cacao are great Paleo treats. Chocolate is an antioxidant and contains healthy minerals. Look for a brand free of soy lecithin if possible, since soy is off the table. Just to be clear, chocolate is a treat, not a meal. Most dessert chocolate contains sugar, so keep your portions small. For baking, use unsweetened chocolate and sweeten with honey.

Dried Fruit is high in natural sugar, so it is best limited to when you need a convenient food to go. Dried fruit also often contains sulfur dioxide as a preservative and/or added sugar so try to buy organic fruit, free of preservatives and added sugar.

White Rice is a grain but one without gluten or anti-nutrients, so have your sushi on occasion. Or just switch to sashimi. Rice does contain anti-nutrients, but they are in the outer shell, which is still present in brown rice, and removed to make white rice.

Quinoa is a seed, but it acts like a grain (called a pseudo grain), containing anti-nutrients, including saponins, which can damage the intestinal wall. Some of the saponins can be "polished" and rinsed off, but quinoa still doesn't rate high in nutrient-density. Avoid eating in large quantity.

Sprouted Legumes can be eaten in moderation. If legumes are soaked until they sprout before cooking, it reduces the anti-nutrients and makes them less irritable to your gut than regular cooked legumes. They still contain anti-nutrients so keep consumption of all legumes to a minimum.

White Potatoes are not recommended in large portions, because they contain anti-nutrients (phytic acid, lectins and saponins) that impair absorption of nutrients. They also have a high glycemic level (high sugar content). But hey, grabbing a fry from someone else's plate is too fun to pass up on occasion. If they are sweet potato fries, you can order your own.

Dairy is highly individual. A large percentage of people have some level of dairy intolerance, so it is best to eliminate dairy for a month when starting Paleo and then re-introduce it. If you don't have any intolerance and want to incorporate dairy into your diet, go for it! Best are organic, full-fat (which has more nutrients than low-fat) products from grass-fed, happy cows. Raw unprocessed dairy direct from a farmer retains all its nutrients but is difficult to source for most people. Fewer people have aversions to goat or sheep dairy than cow dairy so those are a good choice. Fermented dairy or cultured dairy products (yogurt, kefir, cheese, sour cream) are easier on the gut because the lactose is destroyed during fermentation. Many fermented dairy products also offer probiotic benefits.

Vegetable Juice is okay in moderation, but the fiber in whole vegetables helps slow down the release of sugars and feeds the good bacteria in your gut. Whenever possible, eat your food, don't drink it. When you need a veggie boost and can't find enough fresh food, drink green juice containing things like kale and spinach and avoid ones that contain high amounts of fruit juice.

Smoothies that include some fat (avocado or nut butter) and some protein (yogurt or kefir) are okay once in a while. Fruit smoothies are not meal replacements, as they contain almost all carbs. If you are going to drink smoothies, use low-sugar fruits (berries) and try to add some greens to it.

Kombucha is fermented tea that can be beneficial to gut health. It is made with sugar, so it is a bit controversial, but in moderation it seems the positives outweigh the negatives.

soaking legumes

1. RINSE

2. PLACE in a glass BOWL OR POT

3. COVER with warm, filtered water + pinch of BAKING SODA

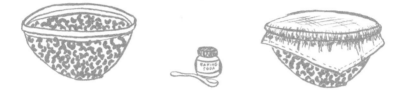

4. FOR every cup of liquid add 1 TBSP. OF ACidic Medium

5. COVER with a clean TOWEL + RUBBER-BAND

6. Soak for 12-24 hours, changing WATER + Baking soda ONCE OR TWICE

7. RINSE

8. REPLACE WATER and cook FOR 4-8 hours on low heat UNTILL BEANS are tender

Note:

yogurt & buttermilk are common 'acidic mediums'

Alcohol is okay to have sometimes. Not too much. Preferably wine, tequila or hard cider, since those alcohols are not made from grains.

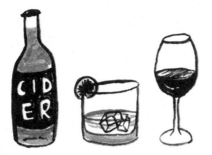

Use for Cooking and Flavor

Honey or Maple Syrup are the best sweeteners. Molasses, coconut sugar, palm sugar, stevia and quite a few others are mentioned as acceptable by some Paleo chefs. One thing is clear, they are all still sugar, so use sparingly.

Butter, Ghee, Coconut Oil, Olive Oil, Animal Fats (lard or duck fat) and occasionally cold-pressed avocado or nut oils are all healthy fats for cooking.

Vinegar and Fruit Juice are good acids for cooking and can be used to flavor foods. Fruit juices, including citrus, have high levels of sugar in the form of fructose that can be quickly released in your system due to the relatively low amount of fiber, so they are only recommended as flavor additives, not beverages.

Nut and Coconut Flours can be used as Paleo substitutes for grain flour in cooking. Almond flour is most common and consists of finely ground almonds. Coconut flour is the dried and ground meat of coconuts. See the cooking section of this book for more Paleo flour options.

Off the Table

Grains—including wheat, barley, rye, oats, spelt, corn—and pseudo grains (plant seeds that act like grains) buckwheat and amaranth all contain anti-nutrients. Anti-nutrients are compounds—like phytic acid, lectin, and saponins—that are found in foods and interfere with the absorption of nutrients. They also break down your intestinal wall, allowing food particles and other toxins to "leak" out of your intestine and into your bloodstream where they do not belong, causing "leaky gut" and resulting in inflammation. White rice and the pseudo grain quinoa can be consumed in little amounts because they seem to be considered neutral in terms of nutrient-density.

Corn is a grain. It is also full of sugar and starch, not to mention the genetic modification of much corn. Just say no to corn. And watch the documentary films *Food, Inc* and *King Corn* to learn more about corn.

Gluten is the protein in some grains that provides the elasticity in foods and holds them together. Remember when you mixed white flour and water as a kid to make glue? Some of the kids ate it, and it was fine. But would you want to eat glue now? Gluten = Glue. If you wonder why you often feel bloated or constipated, try eliminating the glue from your food. By eliminating all grains, you eliminate gluten.

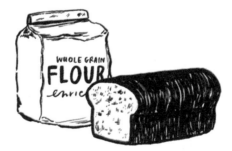

Bread usually contains gluten. Gluten-free bread does not mean free of grain, so it is still off the table. If indulging in a bite of fresh-baked bread slathered in butter is your vice of choice, don't do it too often and don't waste that bite on anything less than greatness. If you have access to bread made by natural fermentation from high-nutrient, hand-milled grains, those products would be likely be considered nutrient dense and Paleo friendly in small amounts.

Pasta contains grains. Try substituting zucchini pasta, which is deliciously satisfying and still holds the pasta sauce for you.

Legumes contain anti-nutrients (phytic acid, which binds to nutrients preventing absorption, and saponins and lectins, which damage the intestinal wall.) Almost everything ending in bean or pea is a no (excluding fresh green beans and peas, coffee beans, vanilla beans and cocoa beans) and including chickpeas and lentils. However, if you are at a potluck and they run out of everything else that is Paleo, a small portion of legumes isn't the worst thing for you.

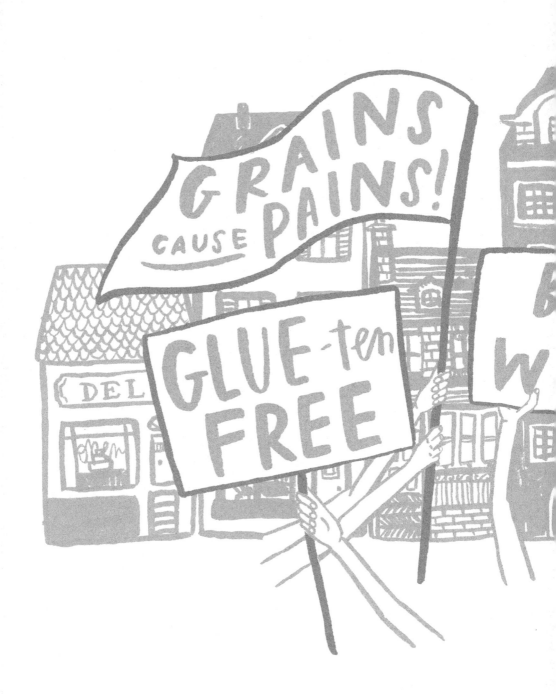

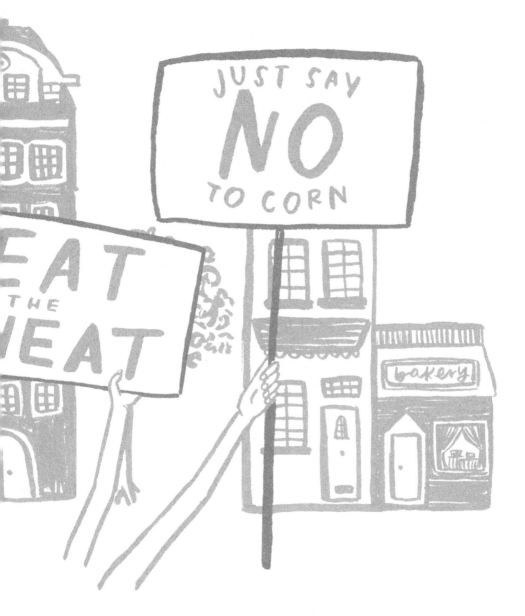

Peanuts are not nuts; they are legumes. Sometimes it seems like a nut, but it's not. So if you feel like a nut, eat a real nut.

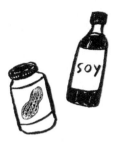

Soy is another legume worth mentioning. Just to be clear, no tofu, no soy milk, no miso, no nothing that is a soybean product. In addition to the fact that it contains the same lectins and phytic acid as other legumes, soy also contains phytoestrogens that mimic estrogen in the body, causing hormonal problems.

Soy Sauce is made from soy (a legume), and it also contains gluten. If you are a sushi or sashimi addict and want your soy sauce, ask for Tamari, which is a Japanese soy product without the gluten, so at least you eliminate one of the non-Paleo ingredients. Or substitute coconut aminos, a soy-free seasoning sauce that is Paleo.

Processed Food typically contains preservatives and is presented in a package. Preservatives are meant to inhibit bacterial growth and those preservatives can also inhibit the good bacteria in your body that keep your gut healthy and help you properly digest your food. You can find packaged foods (like frozen fruits and vegetables) that are free of preservatives, but proceed with caution and always check ingredient labels.

Refined Sugar is the white stuff that comes in a bag or box. Or the brown stuff in the bag or box. Most of the time you can substitute honey, maple syrup or fruit juice. Look up recipes for Paleo desserts if this concerns you. You need not worry that you will never eat dessert again.

Candy is made primarily of refined sugar. Just say goodbye to Mr. Goodbar. Handmade, artisanal, dark chocolates made from superior products can be enjoyed in moderation.

Refined Oils including margarine, corn oil, peanut oil, canola oil, safflower oil, grapeseed oil and many others use chemicals or heat to extract the oil, destroying any nutrients they might have had. Substitute these with butter, ghee, coconut oil, olive oil, animal fats (lard or duck fat) or occasionally cold-pressed avocado or nut oils.

Soda, Soft Drinks, Energy Drinks and anything resembling drinks that contain sugar or artificial sweeteners are off the table. No more needs to be said on that subject.

Beer is made from fermented grains so it is a no, unless you have been really, really good on everything else and it is a super hot day. Even then, just drink tequila with sparkling water or a glass of wine or hard cider instead of beer.

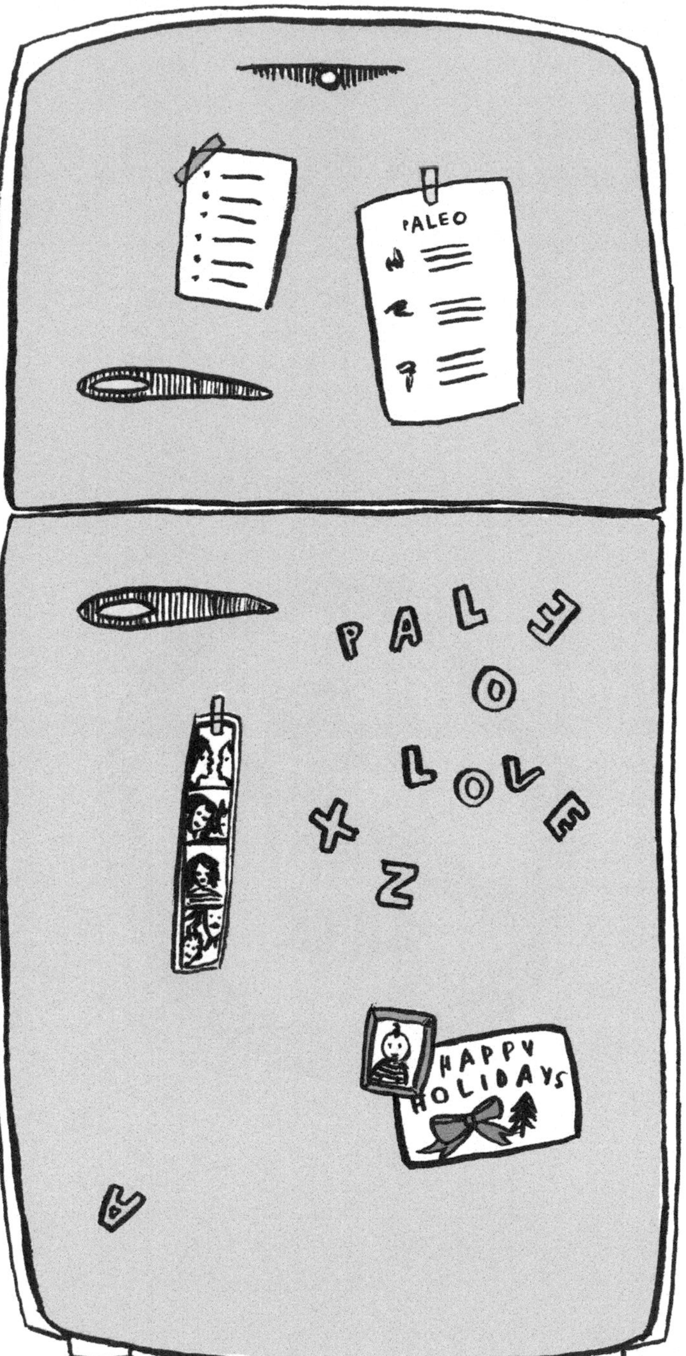
PALEO
PALEO
LOVE
X
Z
HAPPY HOLIDAYS

The Paleo
CHEAT SHEET

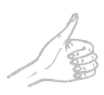

Vegetables
Animal Protein
Fruits
Fermented Foods
Healthy Fats & Oils

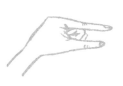

Chocolate
Nuts & Seeds
Gluten-free starches
Honey & Maple Syrup
Alcohol

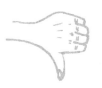

Grains
Legumes
Dairy
Sugar
Processed Foods
Vegetable & Seed Oils

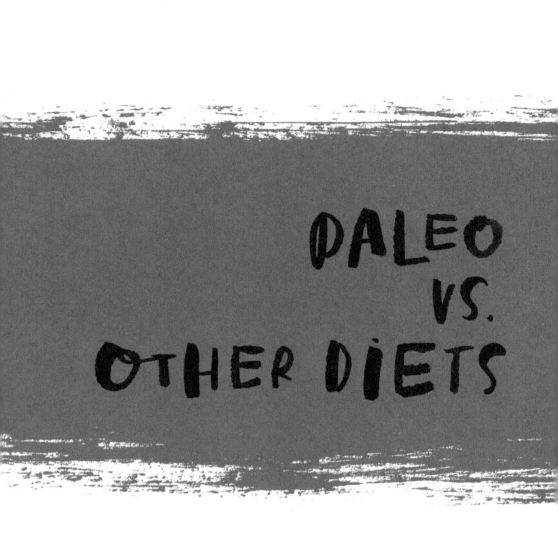

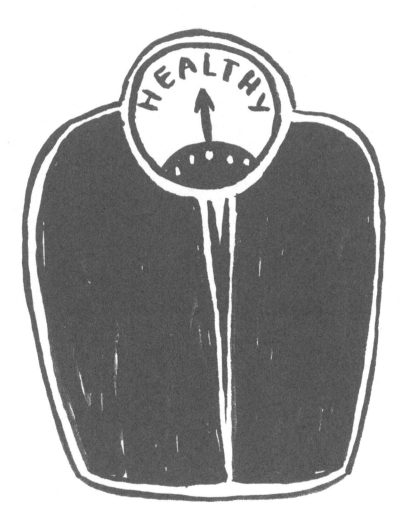

How does Paleo differ from Atkins & other low-carbohydrate diets?

Paleo guidelines have been developed and interpreted by people interested in optimal health, and there is not one absolute structure. Atkins, South Beach and other commercial diets were primarily created for weight loss and are very structured, with specific meal plans and the ability to purchase convenience foods. While they are high protein, these diets typically include dairy, legumes and grains with careful programming of allowances.

How does Paleo differ from Primal?

Some sources define Primal as Paleo that includes dairy. Some say Primal also includes limited legumes. Others don't make any distinctions and use the terms interchangeably.

Paleo and Primal are like hunter-gatherer brothers. They all live in harmony in the same type of cave, hunting in the same forest. One brother loves cheese and another can't live without peas, but they are part of one big, healthy, protein-loving family.

Paleo and Primal are also described as Ancestral, Caveman, and Hunter-Gatherer. None of these diets are commercial, meaning no one owns the idea or meal plans, and they are therefore variable and open to interpretation.

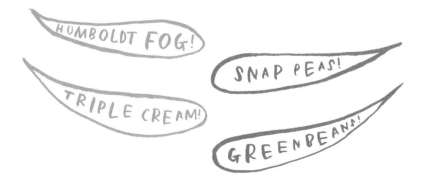

Can I be Paleo & vegetarian?

Short answer is yes. If you are willing to put in the effort, it can be done. It is difficult to be strictly vegetarian and Paleo, but with some careful research and planning, you can find a balance that works for you. Please be sure to do your research before beginning, because you may find yourself lacking in many essential nutrients if you do not plan ahead and map out your nutrient sources. Some tips are:

- *Be sure to find an alternate source of essential Omega-3 fatty acids. Flaxseed and flaxseed oil are high in Omega-3s.*

- *Eat ample whole eggs to help fill the protein gap.*

- *Add to your protein with quinoa, which is an "Eat Little" food from the Paleo Table.*

- *Eat soaked and sprouted legumes for protein. While legumes are not typically recommended, soaking and/or sprouting them is said to decrease the effects of the anti-nutrients.*

What about Paleo & vegan?

There are people who say it can be done. But since nutrient-dense animal protein is a mainstay of the Paleo diet, vegan Paleo isn't really Paleo anymore, is it?

COMMON QUESTIONS ABOUT PALEO

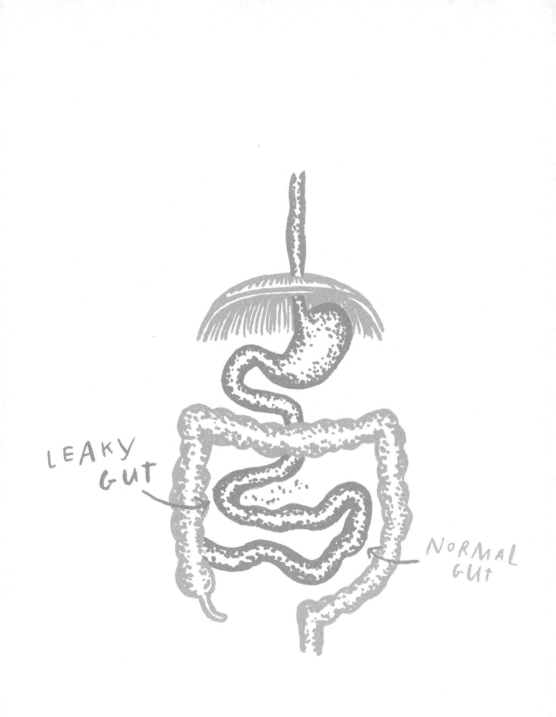

LEAKY GUT

NORMAL GUT

What are anti-nutrients?

Anti-nutrients are compounds—like phytic acid, lectin and saponins—found in foods, and they interfere with the absorption of nutrients. They also break down your intestinal wall, allowing food particles and other toxins to "leak" out of your intestine and into your bloodstream, where they do not belong (causing "leaky gut.") Your immune system senses these foreign substances in the bloodstream and goes into attack mode, producing antibodies that can attack your healthy cells, lead to allergies and, some believe, autoimmune diseases. Some anti-nutrients are lessened with cooking and even more so with soaking and sprouting, as in the case of grains and legumes.

What does inflammation have to do with it?

Inflammation is your body's response to an injury. It is basically your immune system sending help. Your body needs acute inflammation to allow injuries to heal and protect them from infection. But chronic inflammation can lead to a host of physical problems. Stress and lack of sleep are contributors to chronic inflammation. So are a variety of foods like grains and legumes, which contain anti-nutrients that cause "leaky gut" and send your immune system signals that trigger inflammation. Paleo stresses eating a minimal amount of these inflammation-causing foods to avoid chronic inflammation.

What's a leaky gut?

Foods like legumes and grains contain anti-nutrients that can increase the permeability of your intestinal wall. This means that food particles and other toxins "leak" out of your intestine and into your bloodstream. Your immune system senses these foreign substances in the bloodstream and produces antibodies which can attack your healthy cells and lead to allergies. Some medical professionals believe that autoimmune diseases can begin with "leaky gut."

Why no legumes?

Legumes contain phytic acid, which prevents you from absorbing all the nutrients in the legumes so they can't be considered a nutrient-dense food. Even after soaking and cooking to minimize the anti-nutrients, legumes still aren't dense in nutrients. They also contain lectins, which damage your intestinal wall. Small amounts of legumes aren't the worst thing to eat on occasion if you can't live without "Beans, Beans, the Magical Fruit."

What is acid & alkaline balance?

Foods register in your body as either acid-forming (dairy, grains, most legumes, most animal protein) or alkaline-forming (most fruits and vegetables, some nuts). If your diet is acid heavy, it pulls calcium from your bones to bring it back to balance, therefore causing bone de-mineralization and poor bone health. Eating Paleo promotes acid and alkaline balance by recommending fresh fruits and vegetables daily with no grains or legumes. Be careful to keep your animal protein intake (acid) in balance by eating lots of fruits and vegetables (alkaline).

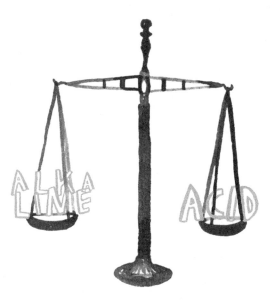

If early man ate grains, why can't we?

Early man ate wild or cultivated-from wild grains that were full of nutrients. Preparing the grains was very labor-intensive, involving hand-harvesting, toasting and pounding to make a digestible paste. The quantities would have been small and very nutritious, unlike almost all grain products today. If you are lucky enough to have access to high-nutrient, hand-milled grains, and breads made by natural fermentation of those grains, those products would be considered nutrient dense and Paleo friendly in small amounts.

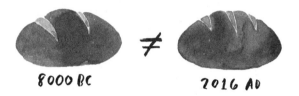

8000 BC ≠ 2016 AD

How do I get fiber without grains?

A typical day of eating Paleo should include plenty of fiber in the form of vegetables, fruits, nuts and seeds.

What if I get carb cravings?

Most people mean pasta and bread when they say carb cravings. Those cravings come from your old way of eating, which didn't provide for stable blood sugar levels and didn't allow for fully satisfying meals that include proteins and fats. Out of habit, you may initially struggle to avoid certain foods. But your body should not crave them once you adjust to Paleo. Give yourself a month of eating Paleo, and the cravings will likely disappear.

Can I eat gluten-free bread?

Bread usually contains grains even if it is gluten free. If bread is your vice and that's what you need to get started being Paleo, then try to find one made with rice flour and freshly baked with quality ingredients. You can find Paleo breads in some places, but they might be packed with high-calorie nut flours, so eat all bread sparingly.

Should athletes eat more carbs?

The amount of carbohydrates you need to function optimally on the Paleo diet is highly individualized. Athletes and people with high daily exertion levels tend to need more carbohydrates in their daily intake. But that does not mean pasta and bread! Plenty of Paleo foods contain carbohydrates. Starchy vegetables like sweet potatoes, squash, beets and carrots are the highest in carbs. Fruits like apples, pears, bananas and grapes are filled with carbs but are also higher in sugar in the form of fructose. Dried fruits like dates and raisins are very high carb and very high sugar. Try to find the right balance of carbohydrates for your lifestyle, still keeping your sugar levels at a minimum.

What are starchy foods and are they ALL bad?

Starchy foods are high in carbohydrates with a complex molecular sugar structure that contains a large number of glucose units. Tuber vegetables—like potatoes and yams—and all grains are considered "starchy." The body needs glucose to function, but glucose is also produced in the body so there are differing opinions on the optimal level of starchy foods to ingest. Paleo recommends eating minimal amounts of non-grain starch like sweet potatoes. High-intensity athletes may need moderate levels of starchy foods.

Why sweet potatoes but not white potatoes?

Both are carbohydrates with a high glycemic index (which means they have a large effect on blood sugar level), but sweet potatoes have more beneficial nutrients than white potatoes and do not contain the anti-nutrients saponin and lectin that white potatoes contain. Non-processed, white potatoes without the skin (which also contains anti-nutrients) can be eaten on occasion.

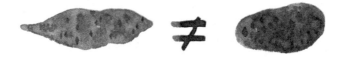

Why white rice, not brown?

Most of the anti-nutrients found in rice are contained in the outer shell. While brown rice may have nutrients that white rice does not, they are not absorbed well because of the anti-nutrients. That outer shell is removed in white rice, taking away the anti-nutrients, making white rice nutrient neutral.

What is grass-fed & pasture-raised?

You are not *just* what you eat. As Michael Pollan so insightfully stated, "You are what you eat eats." Animals from large-scale feed lots can be grain fed or grain finished to quickly fatten them up for processing. Cows are meant to eat grass (grass fed), not grains. Chickens and pigs are natural foragers so they should be allowed to forage freely in pastures (pasture raised.) Many smaller farms have adopted this concept, and we are finding grass-fed and pastured products becoming increasingly available both in stores and online.

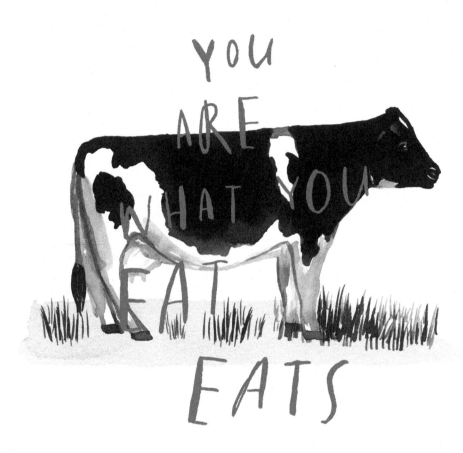

YOU ARE WHAT YOU EAT EATS

-MICHAEL POLLAN
In Defense of Food:
An Eater's Manifesto

Is BACON Paleo?

Well-sourced bacon from pasture-raised pigs, containing no added ingredients except salt and spices, is Paleo. Most available bacon does not reach these standards so check labels carefully.

Isn't red meat bad for me?

Information in the press tells us that meat contains carcinogens, which is certainly alarming to read. However, if you drill down to the real facts, there is little reality in these statements when it pertains to moderate consumption of grass-fed and pasture-raised products. The research seems to be based on people who eat grain-fed meat, fast food and/or processed meat products. And even then, it seems that the studies don't typically isolate what else these people are consuming.

What about cholesterol?

What about it? Scientific research suggests that eating high-cholesterol food does not raise blood cholesterol levels (except for a small increase in people known as hyper-responders) and does not increase your risk of heart disease. Cholesterol is a necessary molecule involved with hormones, the immune system and the brain. It plays only a minor role in heart disease. Inflammation is thought to be the primary cause of heart disease.

Can I have green drinks & smoothies?

If you have trouble keeping on weight or don't have regular access to fresh produce, adding a vegetable drink to your diet can be helpful. For the rest of us, adding these calories that are quickly absorbed without the benefit of fiber, is unnecessary. In the case of fruit drinks that don't contain added fat or protein (from avocado or nut butter), the sugars are digested quickly and can cause problems with blood glucose levels if juice becomes a daily habit.

Are protein drinks okay?

Protein powder, consumed in the form of a drink, is only recommended as a calorie supplement for an extreme athlete. They are not effective meal replacements unless you really need the convenience and you are very confident with the source of the product. The ingredients in protein powders are not regulated in the United States because they are supplements, not food. Therefore, you really don't know what you are getting in your processed package. There can also be a problematic insulin response caused by protein drinks, but that is too much science to go into here. Google it. Right after you throw out your enormous tub of protein powder.

What if I lose too much weight?

If you adhere very strictly to a Paleo regime while maintaining a strenuous workout schedule, you may have trouble keeping on weight while adjusting to Paleo and discovering what foods work for you. If you go below your desired weight, add extra carbohydrates in the form of sweet potatoes and fruits, along with plenty of protein. Add dairy and/or protein shakes (from reputable sources) if desired.

Do I need supplements?

You shouldn't need an arsenal of supplements when consistently eating nutrient-dense meals including animal proteins and organically grown fruits and vegetables. However, vitamin and mineral needs are highly personal and in today's world—even eating Paleo—it is sometimes difficult to get the full complement of nutrients. Vitamin D is a particular problem, especially if you work inside all day and do not get regular exposure to sun. Check with a medical expert to determine what supplements may be good for your specific lifestyle.

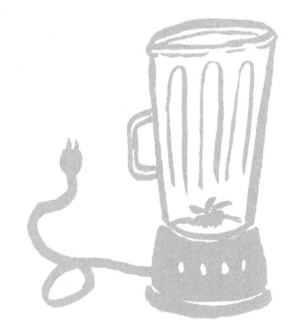

EAT YOUR FOOD,

don't drink it.

Are bone marrow & bone broth essential?

Bone marrow and bone broth contain nutrients like collagen, glucosamine and gelatin that are difficult to find elsewhere. Bone marrow is mostly fat and nutrients. The marrow and broth are both highly nutritious and most Paleo enthusiasts strongly advocate the health benefits. If you are having any digestive or stomach problems, bone broth can help. You can purchase grass-fed bone broth online or make it yourself by roasting, then boiling meat bones for many hours before straining the broth.

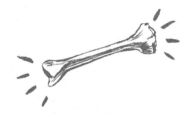

What is offal? (and is it AWFUL?)

Offal is the edible, non-skeletal-muscle parts of an animal, including but not limited to the liver, heart, feet, tongue and brains. Although not hugely popular in the United States, many other countries treasure these nutrient-dense parts of the animal that fall when the meat is butchered, or literally "off-fall" the carcass.

What are nightshades?

Paleo is often recommended for people with autoimmune diseases and the topic of nightshades then arises. Nightshades are a plant family that can cause joint pain and inflammation in people who are sensitive to them. They include eggplant, tomatoes, peppers and potatoes among other plants and are in a wide variety of condiments like hot sauce and spices including paprika. It is suggested that anyone with an autoimmune disease avoid nightshades.

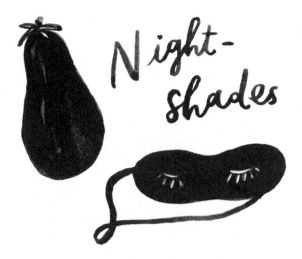

Night-shades

How do fermented foods fit in?

Fermented foods are probiotic, which means they contain bacteria that aid the health of your gut. Check the labels to be sure your fermented products (like pickles and sauerkraut) only contain Paleo-friendly ingredients and are raw and unpasteurized. It is also very easy to ferment your own vegetables with just salt and water. Kombucha is a fermented tea that is approved by many Paleo enthusiasts, even though it is fermented with sugar because the positives outweigh the negatives. If you eat dairy, yogurt is also a fermented product.

Can I use condiments?

Condiments may contain sugar, artificial sweeteners, soy, wheat or refined oils, among other ingredients. Anything you cannot pronounce is probably not Paleo! However, if you are only eating a teaspoon a month, it may not be noteworthy in your overall diet. If there is a condiment you love and eat with significant frequency, take the time to look at the ingredients. You may choose to find a Paleo brand or a recipe to make a Paleo version of it.

The LIFESTYLE

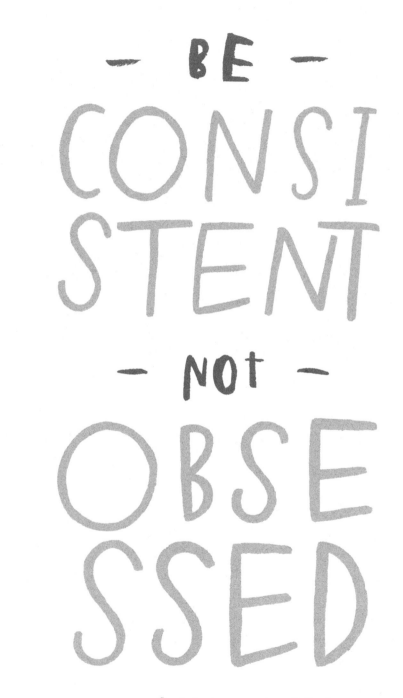

BE

CONSI
STENT

NOT

OBSE
SSED

THE #1 RULE of PALEO

What is the NUMBER ONE rule of Paleo?

Be consistent, not obsessed. Everyone's lifestyle and food preferences are different. What works for your Paleo friend may not work for you. Don't let perfection get in the way of your best health. If you feel great ending your meal with some cheese and apple slices, then have it! Work within the Paleo guidelines, and discover what is best for you.

Is Paleo expensive?

Some Paleo-preferred foods, like grass-fed beef and organic produce can be more expensive. However, nutrient per dollar, you will come out ahead. It costs more to buy eggs and fresh fruit for breakfast than a Pop-Tart. But you won't be hungry two hours after breakfast, and you won't need as many visits to your doctor. While it might take some planning and home cooking, you can eat Paleo quite well on a budget. There are online resources and even budget Paleo cookbooks to guide you toward effective meal planning.

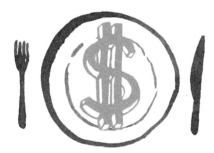

Is Paleo healthy for children?

Babies love mashed banana and avocado. Children thrive on non-processed, fresh, whole foods. Paleo is a healthy diet for people of all ages. As with any diet, foods should be introduced to young children one at a time to test for sensitivities or allergies, and all children should receive regular medical checkups to ensure they are receiving the nutrition they need to properly develop.

Will Paleo make me constipated?

Some people think that Paleo will not work for them because they can't poop when they eat a lot of meat. It probably isn't the meat that is blocking them up, but what they eat with the meat.

Think of a typical barbecue with friends. It starts with chips and dip. Meat is paired with a bun or garlic bread. With corn on the cob and potatoes or beans, your meal is a gluten and carbohydrate feast.

Compare that to the Paleo plate for a BBQ. You begin with dip and raw veggies. You have a salad, lots of vegetables and a piece of meat. The Paleo meal, with its fiber and lack of gluten, is better designed to keep your system regular. You should have no trouble pooping.

Are there times of day to eat certain foods?

Timing rules, such as you should always eat fruit in the morning or only have protein for dinner, are restrictions that belong more to other types of diets. Protein and good fats should be eaten at every meal if possible, combined with a daily balance of carbs.

How much do I eat of what?

Each meal should contain a protein portion about the size of your palm along with vegetables, fruits and healthy fats. You likely won't be hungry between meals unless you are very active. If you do find yourself hungry between meals, you can eat as many snacks as you like, as long as you stick to the foods on the Paleo Table.

How can I SURVIVE giving up so many foods?

Being Paleo 80 percent of the time will yield fantastic results for you and your health. That means every day you could eat something that is on the Eat Little list. You could have sushi or a glass of wine or ice cream. You should avoid having all three in the same day, but if you do, get right back on track the next day. The most important thing is to be consistent, not obsessed.

Should I avoid packaged products labeled Paleo?

Misinformation suggests that Paleo is about eating only what was available in Paleolithic times. The authentic Paleo lifestyle incorporates foods that support the idea of a nutrient-dense diet. Modern products like Paleo Mayonnaise, Baobab Powder and Grain-free Granola will continue to enter the market and will be perfectly acceptable to the Paleo community. The important thing is to look at the ingredients to decide if it fits into your Paleo guidelines.

Can I still drink alcohol?

If you want to raise a glass with friends, that can be part of your Paleo diet. Wine, tequila or hard cider are the most Paleo-friendly alcohols, because they are not made from grains.

Does Paleo affect libido?

Many factors go into a healthy sex drive, so no one can claim that eating Paleo in and of itself will affect libido. However, if Paleo works for you, it should be affecting the way you look and the way you feel. Whether the result is newfound confidence, balanced hormones or corrected nutritional deficiencies, enthusiasts claim that eating Paleo improves life in and out of the bedroom!

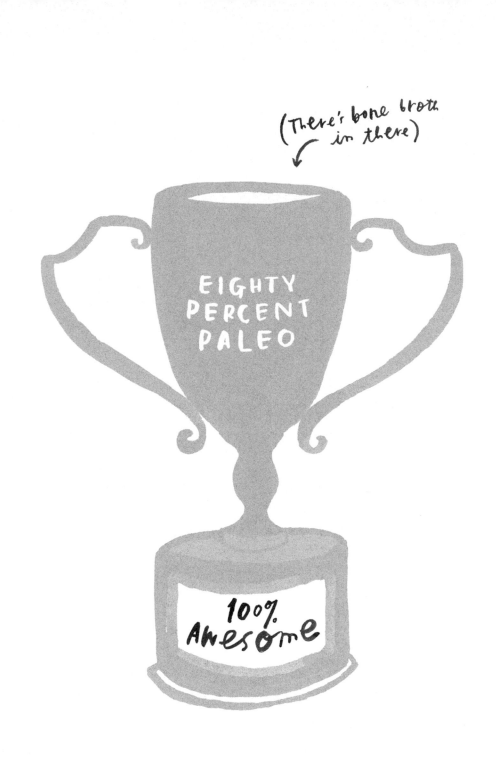

Do I HAVE to exercise to be Paleo?

No. But you will probably want to. The great news is that once you start eating mostly Paleo, your energy should increase and your outlook improve. Suddenly, going for a run or hitting the gym will sound like fun. Well...if you are afraid of exercise, it may not sound fun, but you will at least feel like it is better than going to the dentist.

What's the DEAL with Crossfit?

CrossFit is a type of intense workout that has become very popular in recent years, and many CrossFit athletes believe in eating Paleo. You will likely find a supportive and welcoming Paleo community at a CrossFit gym. Most gyms have a free trial, so it is worth going to see if CrossFit is something you might enjoy. It is based on the concept of the hunter-gatherer lifestyle of carrying heavy things, running, climbing and jumping. Sounds like fun!

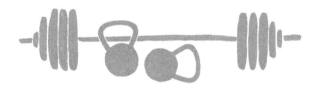

How is SLEEP involved?

Paleo enthusiasts are big proponents of at least seven hours of sleep per night for overall well-being. Experts suggest that lack of sleep can increase your cravings for non-Paleo foods, because lack of sleep has an effect on the hormones affecting appetite control.

Why is sunlight a factor?

Sunlight is another contributor of the Paleolithic model of food, exercise, sleep, and sunlight. Sunlight elevates levels of vitamin D, which is a very important vitamin for good health. While vitamin D is present in foods, it is very difficult to get enough from diet alone, so try to get 15-20 minutes or more of sunshine a day to increase your vitamin D levels. Sunscreen blocks the ability to create the vitamin D, so you need to soak in the rays before putting on sunscreen. Vitamin D is also available in supplement form.

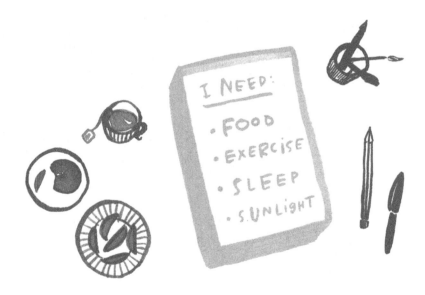

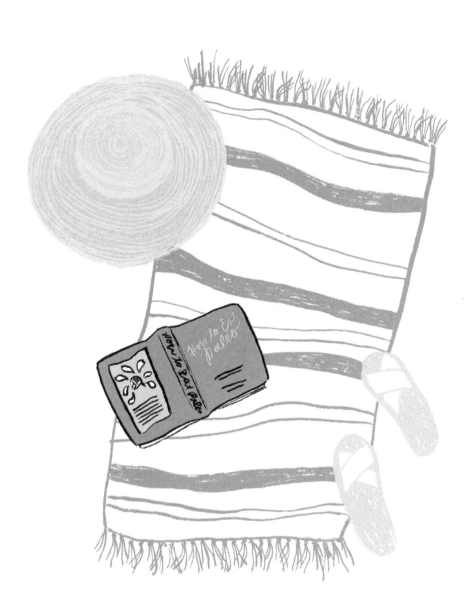

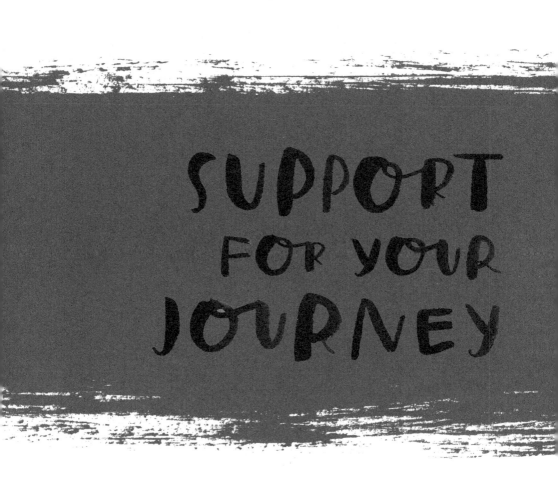

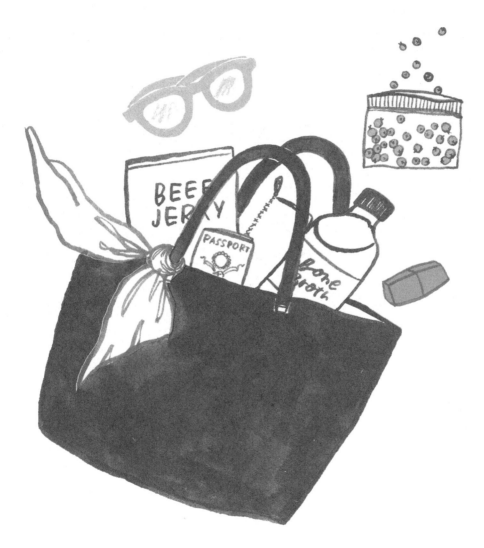

Common Misconceptions

We Only Eat
What a Caveman Ate

Ridiculous. There were no chickens free-ranging in the Stone Age. Paleo foods are chosen because of the nutrient density that attempts to mimic the nutritional characteristics of foods from Paleolithic times. That time existed before large-scale agriculture and farming created innovations, some of which, have resulted in foods with less nutritional value.

We Often Make a Meal of
a Big Plate of Meat

No! Never! We don't live in caves and are not hunting for our food so there is no reason to limit ourselves to the "kill" of the day. Meat is one type of protein that we eat, and the protein on our plate should always be balanced with plenty of fresh produce.

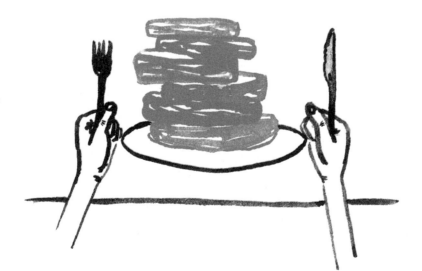

We Cannot Eat Out at Restaurants
Because Our Diet Is Too Limiting

Not true! Aside from vegetarian and vegan establishments, restaurants always have animal protein and vegetables on the menu. Eating out is a joy.

We Can't Attend Dinner Parties
Because We Can't Eat the Food

Completely false! Eating Paleo is no different than being gluten free or vegetarian or having any other dietary choice when going to a dinner party. If the hosts ask about diet, you can gratefully give them the easy answer of "We love all fish, meat and poultry, as well as salad, vegetables and fruit." If you know them well, you can add, "We are gluten free so we don't eat pasta or bread." If the hostess doesn't ask about your diet, offer to bring a dish! Or just hope the meal includes some form of protein and vegetables, which it usually does, so eat as Paleo-ish as you can.

We Have to Travel With All Our Own Food
Because There Is No Paleo Food in Airports

We may prefer to pack a meal, but it is possible to get by when traveling. Airports and airplanes don't typically have food that any health-conscious person would enjoy eating, but that is beginning to change at some airports.

We Are All
CrossFit Fanatics

There is a large population of the Paleo community that does the popular fitness program called CrossFit. And there are also plenty of Paleo enthusiasts that have never seen a CrossFit gym. If you have a CrossFit gym in your town, check it out! It is a great way to meet Paleo friends and learn more about the lifestyle. You might also get some Paleo recipes and tips for foraging in your neighborhood.

YOU CAN DO THIS!

When something is not understood, it is often ridiculed. Paleo is one of those things. People may make assumptions due to misinformation, and you can choose to inform or ignore them. When you start looking and feeling great, the naysayers won't bother you much and you may decide to start informing the ones that do.

If you are concerned about standing out, don't be! You will not be shunned in your social circles for eating real food, and many people will not even notice if you choose not to tell them. Paleo food is real food, and you can eat lots of it, so it won't look like you are on any type of special diet.

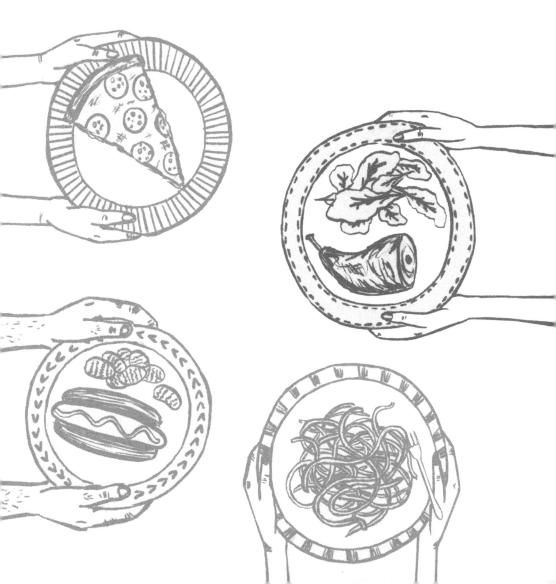

Eating Paleo in a restaurant is simply knowing what to order. Every restaurant has protein and/or vegetables. Even a pizza joint has salad and animal protein toppings.

It is perfectly okay to be Paleo-ish. You are in charge of what you decide to eat. And while there may be Paleo-perfect enthusiasts who preach that you must follow all the rules, it is okay to just lean toward eating Paleo if that is what it takes to get you started. Do your best. Enjoy your meals. Once you lean, you will hopefully start to feel a difference and decide to jump all the way in!

You can have your cake. We all have celebrations and events that are worthy of cake, so go ahead and have your cake and eat it too. It would be good if it were gluten free. Even better if it were Paleo. But until ALL your friends decide to eat Paleo, there will be cake. Have a bite. After you have been Paleo for a while, a bite is all you will want.

Paleo eating—providing protein, fat and fiber at every meal—keeps blood sugar stable, so no more afternoon dips or post-sugar highs.

You do not have to eat pounds of red meat every day to be Paleo. Animal protein is an important part of the recommended Paleo diet, but there are many ways to incorporate animal protein such as eggs, fish and poultry.

Most people who consider themselves Paleo eat Paleo about 80 percent of the time. Part of the philosophy of being Paleo is enjoying your good health and the bounty of delicious food on this planet. That includes enjoying friends and family and gatherings, having a glass (or the occasional three) of alcohol, and not being bound with a ball and chain to dietary choices. The goal of the Paleo lifestyle is to be mostly Paleo every day, making your choices from foods On the Paleo Table and rarely, if ever, from foods that are Off the Table.

You can get started slowly. Eliminate refined sugar, dairy and grains from your diet for 30 days, and you will be amazed at how good you feel.

Eating Paleo is primarily about providing the best healing environment for your body from the inside out, not about lists of Dos and Don'ts. The Paleo Table is presented as a guide to the best foods to eat daily.

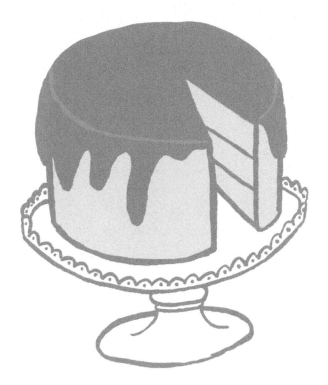

(... YOU KNOW
WHAT TO DO.)

Get OVER it!

The first thing you have to do, as a person new to Paleo, is change your mind-set. We have been programmed to believe certain things about nutrition that are highly controversial. Here are just a few of your new "truths," which can—of course—be disputed by medical experts.

- *Eating fat does not make you fat.*

- *Eating cholesterol does not raise your cholesterol. (Unless you are in the small percentage of people who are hyper-responders to eating cholesterol.)*

- *Eating red meat in moderation will not clog your arteries and cause heart failure. Nor is it a direct cause of cancer.*

- *It is okay to eat a lot if you are hungry.*

- *It is okay to eat eggs every day. Whole eggs.*

- *You don't need to eat whole grains to get enough fiber.*

It is important to eat enough food to fuel your body and mind. Eat breakfast, lunch and dinner. If you haven't eaten in 4-6 hours, plan your next meal even if you aren't yet hungry. If you go too long without eating, you might dive into foods that are not on the Paleo Table like bread or chips.

Paleo is not a weight-loss diet. It is not a plan to drop quick pounds so you will fit into your dress or suit for the big event. It is a way of living. If you decide this is how you are going to eat, you will eventually level out at the ideal weight for your body, losing excess fat where you need to lose it.

THERE'S NO SUCH THING AS *perfect* PALEO.

Tips for traveling away from your cave

You can find Paleo food almost everywhere once you know how to choose. But it is also smart to get an insulated lunch bag for traveling, so you can bring along the foods you prefer.

Airports and airplanes are tough to navigate, as are late nights in small towns. In a real pinch, go to a fast-food restaurant, order a breakfast sandwich or a burger and take it off the bun or ask for a lettuce wrap. It won't be your finest meal, but life on the road isn't always grass-fed beef and organic blueberries. If you need protein and your choices are limited, work with what you have, and don't get completely derailed because of lack of authentic Paleo food choices.

Buy some meat jerky. Jerky is dried meat, so it travels well and lasts throughout a trip. It is also easy to make at home in a regular oven, and you will find wonderfully simple instructions in the recipe section of this book.

Don't forget to prepare for your trip home if you will be gone for a few days! You may not have access to a kitchen or an ice pack, but try to pick up some fresh food before you travel. If that isn't possible, take time to stop and get a protein-filled meal before you get on a plane or train that may not have good Paleo options.

There are many "Paleo" nutrition bars on the market, and new ones are introduced all the time. Some are the real deal and can be a lifesaver when traveling. Choose your bar carefully. Be wary of brands that promote Paleo protein bars and then have peanut butter as a flavor.

Do your best. Grass-fed and pasture-raised products are available but not everywhere. You can source a lot of things through quality grocery stores or local farms. But when you can't, it is okay to make concessions. Buy the best you can, as often as you can.

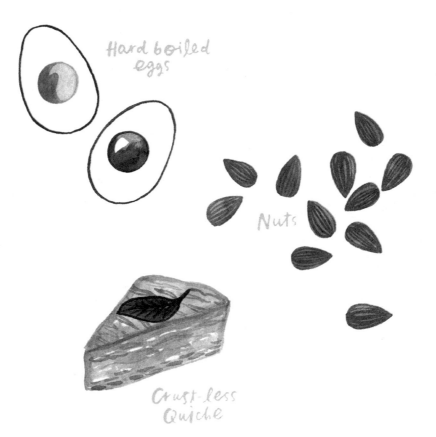

Hard boiled eggs

Nuts

Crust-less Quiche

PALEO
ON the GO

Crudité

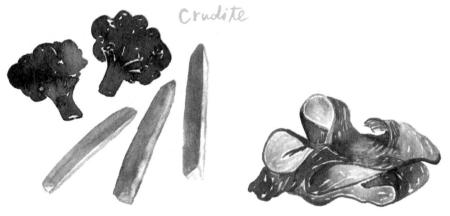

Prosciutto

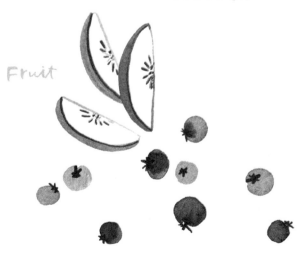

Fruit

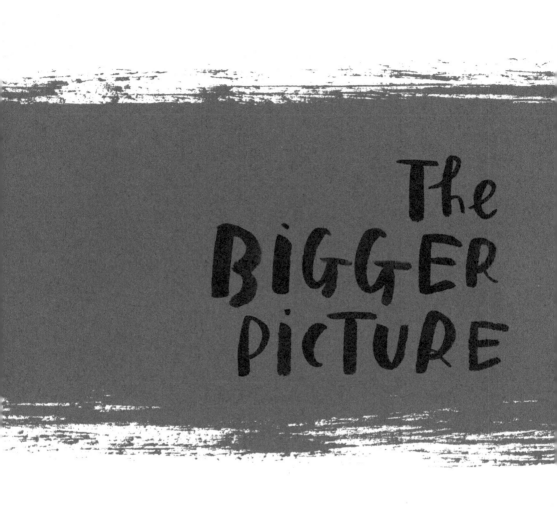

The
BIGGER
PICTURE

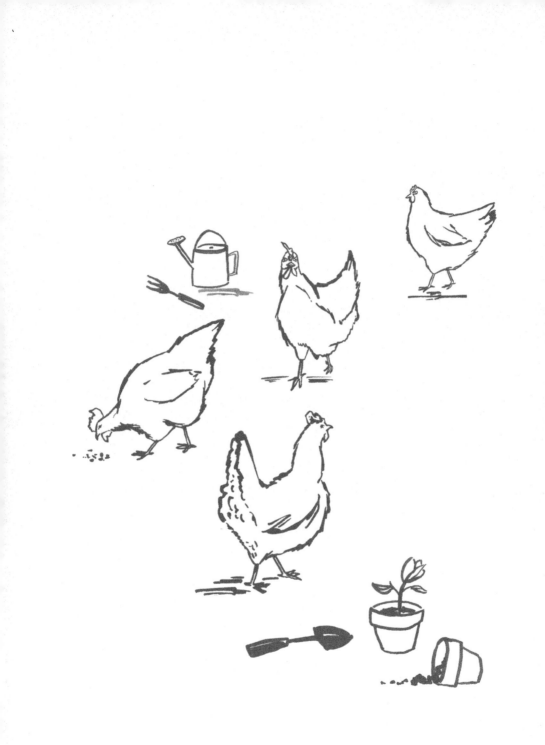

Does Paleo suggest a return to pre-commercial farming techniques?

We don't need to throw away all the modern advances in farming. Our goal is to support the best of farming. If enough people refuse to eat foods with nutrients that have been destroyed through genetic modification and commercial processing, we can open more doors to farmers and artisans who want to use practices resulting in foods with optimal nutrition and taste. Because Paleo has flexible guidelines for eating based on nutritional density, we can evolve our eating as farmers evolve to grow more nutritional offerings.

What's the story on GMOs?

Genetically Modified Organisms (GMOs) are also called Genetically Modified (GM) foods. These GM foods are created by transferring genes from one species of plant or animal to another to create a product with an intended superior quality, like resistance to pests. The problem is that the gene modification can sometimes create unpredictable effects in the food that may cause allergies or nutritional deficiencies.

Are we being environmentally sound by eating Paleo?

It is true that it takes a lot of food and water to create animal protein on a feedlot that feeds cattle grain and uses vast amounts of water to clean them from their own manure and avoid infection. However, small independent farmers are teaching us that livestock have a beneficial role to play as part of an ecology. In other words, in family farms where all the plants and animals live as part of an ecosystem, the livestock are essential to the health of the farm and give (in the form of manure) as much as they take (in the form of grass), so the result is balanced and environmentally sound.

HOW to COOK PALEO

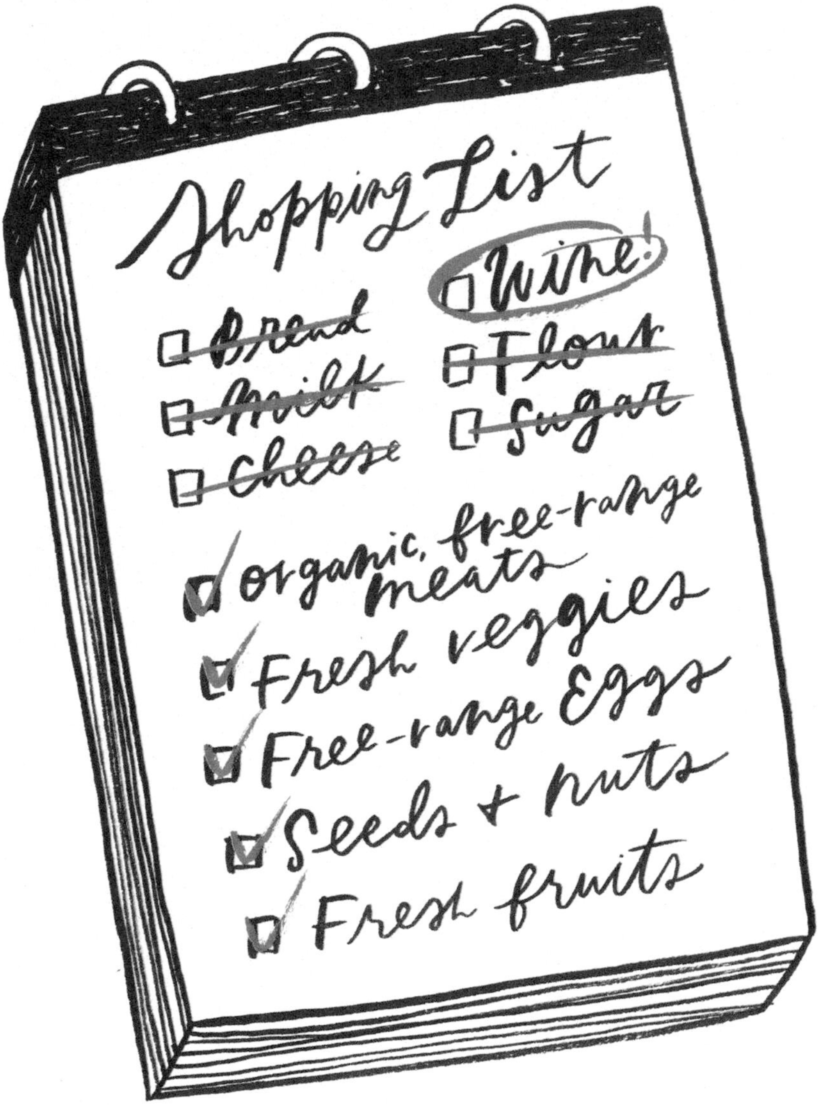

Shopping List

- ☐ ~~Bread~~
- ☐ ~~Milk~~
- ☐ ~~Cheese~~
- ☐ ~~Wine!~~
- ☐ ~~Flour~~
- ☐ ~~Sugar~~

- ☑ organic, free-range meats
- ☑ Fresh veggies
- ☑ Free-range Eggs
- ☑ Seeds + nuts
- ☑ Fresh fruits

Get Started

You don't have to cook to eat Paleo. But eating Paleo involves knowing what you put into your body, so cooking definitely helps control what you eat.

Paleo focuses on fresh, whole ingredients, so feel free to keep it simple and let the foods speak for themselves! Sliced fresh peaches and avocado with olive oil and balsamic vinegar is a treat! Toss it with spinach for a salad. Serve it with a piece of fish or meat and your meal is complete.

Source your ingredients well. Take the time to look around and see what is available to you that is grown nearby. You might need to seek out sources for specialty items like grass-fed beef. There are many farms online that ship frozen meats nationwide.

Cook with natural oils like coconut oil, olive oil, ghee, animal fats (lard or duck) or cold-pressed avocado or nut oils on occasion. If you enjoy dairy products, cook with butter, which is a wonderful, flavorful fat for cooking. Grass-fed or organic butter is available in most areas.

Spices are your friend. They are an inexpensive way to add flavor and variation to simple whole foods.

Check out the abundance of Paleo recipes in cookbooks (like the recipe section included in this book) and online, or find recipes that sound delicious to you and try to make them Paleo.

Experiment! Have fun!

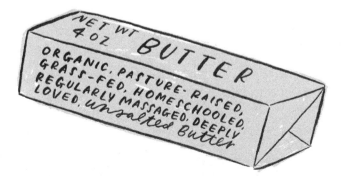

Why no refined oils?

Seeds don't inherently contain a lot of oil, so chemicals or heat are used to extract the oil from the seed. Heat reduces nutrient levels of seed oils and can raise toxicity. It's best to cook with oils cold pressed from olives, coconuts, avocados or nuts. For high-heat cooking, you can use ghee or animal fats like lard or duck fat.

How about flavored oils?

As long as the oil is high-quality cold-pressed oil infused with real ingredients like truffles or herbs, you are good to go. Many flavored oils use artificial "flavoring," so be sure to check the ingredients.

Can I use vinegars?

Yes. Traditionally fermented vinegar (like balsamic or wine vinegar) has probiotic qualities and assists with a healthy gut. However, industrially processed vinegar can contain additives and preservatives that are not Paleo. Purchase good quality, traditionally fermented vinegar with no additives.

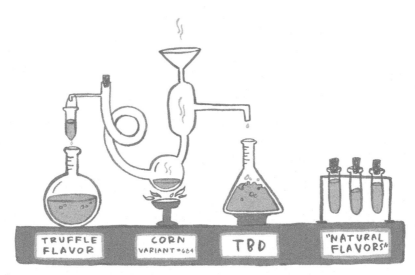

What kind of flour can I use?

There are many flours used in Paleo baking. The most popular are coconut flour, almond flour, tapioca flour and arrowroot flour. Others include sweet potato flour, a variety of nut flours and plantain flour. Most of these flours have different qualities than grain flour (for example, coconut flour adds dryness) so use recipes specific to those flours until you are familiar with how they react. Gluten-free flour blends (which typically contain rice flour and cornstarch) are not recommended unless you find one containing only Paleo-friendly ingredients.

Can I use baking soda & baking powder?

Baking soda is Paleo, and a baking powder substitute can be easily made by mixing 1 part baking soda with 2 parts cream of tartar. Commercial baking powder is not Paleo because it contains ingredients like cornstarch. However, the amount of baking powder used in cooking is minimal so the choice is yours when it comes to purchasing baking powder or making your own.

Is vanilla extract Paleo?

Vanilla extract is Paleo if you choose an extract with no sugar or additives, not a flavoring that is a synthetic, non-Paleo product. Some extracts are made with alcohol distilled from grain, but vanilla is typically used in such minimal amounts it shouldn't make a difference in your diet unless you have an autoimmune disease, in which case you should choose an extract made with grain-free alcohol or make your own.

Isn't agave nectar Paleo?

Agave nectar has higher fructose levels than refined sugar and is highly processed. Honey is a more Paleo option.

Is it okay to salt my food?

Salt is fine as long as you are not salt sensitive, which may cause blood pressure to rise.

Can I cook with soy sauce?

Soy sauce and gluten-free tamari are soy-based products that are not recommended. The Paleo substitute for soy sauce is coconut aminos, which is readily available and bottled very similarly to soy sauce.

Are herbs and spices Paleo?

All herbs and spices—fresh and dried—are great. Eating Paleo is about delicious, well-sourced, well-prepared foods, so make them as flavorful as you like! Check ingredient labels if purchasing prepared mixes or flavorings like hot sauce to ensure they are Paleo friendly if you plan to use them frequently. If you have an autoimmune disease, stay away from nightshades, which include things like paprika and cayenne pepper.

How to throw a
PALEO DINNER PARTY

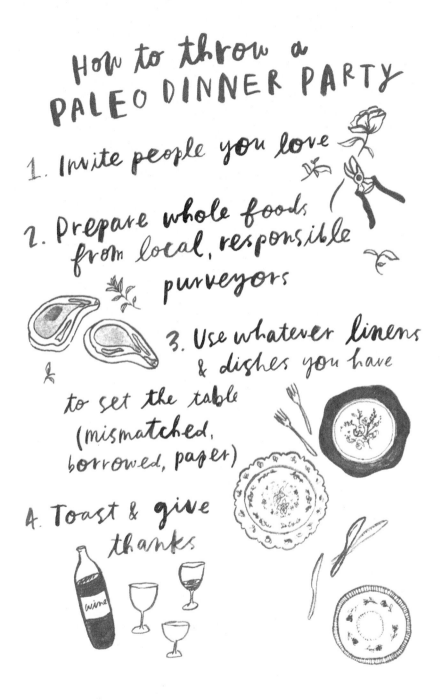

1. Invite people you love

2. Prepare whole foods from local, responsible purveyors

3. Use whatever linens & dishes you have to set the table (mismatched, borrowed, paper)

4. Toast & give thanks

RECIPES

The Paleo community is lucky to have talented chefs creating a constant supply of Paleo recipes. But to eat well with Paleo, you don't need to limit yourself to recipes carrying the Paleo label. Delicious Paleo recipes can be found in all types of cookbooks and from all types of people. The recipes assembled here, contributed by a diverse group of accomplished family and friends, range from party-worthy brunch dishes to simple family fare. Some of the contributors eat Paleo as a lifestyle choice, but most do not. They all enjoy eating real food, so they didn't have to dig too deep into their files to find a favorite recipe that happens to be Paleo. Enjoy!

Recipes & Contributors

Kendall's Beef Jerky

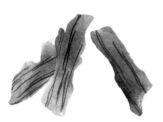

Kendall Conrad is a former model and actress who rides horses, cooks like a chef and is the designer of the Los Angeles-based, luxury accessories brand Kendall Conrad, offering leather goods and jewelry. She is the author of Eat Well Feel Well, *a cookbook designed to manage digestive conditions through eating delicious, healthy food.*

Kendall's Beef Jerky

1 pound grass-fed top sirloin, sliced paper thin by a butcher while slightly frozen (or with a mandolin)

¼ cup extra-virgin olive oil

2 cloves garlic, minced

1 teaspoon salt or to taste

½ teaspoon cayenne pepper

¼ teaspoon ground black pepper

Preheat oven to 175°F.

In a large bowl, mix all ingredients together, coating the meat slices well.

Place the meat slices individually in one layer on baking pans and place in the oven. Leave in the oven 7 to 9 hours until the meat is dried but still a little chewy. Cool completely and store in sealed container in the refrigerator for up to 1 week.

Val's Pickled Cauliflower

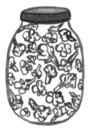

Valerie Rice is an avid cook, gardener and host with a signature California style. Val authors a popular lifestyle blog, Eat-Drink-Garden, *where she encourages readers to live life deliciously! Her witty wisdom is shared nationwide in places like* Sunset Magazine *and* Access Hollywood Live, *where she divulges her best tips, recipes and entertaining recommendations on living the good life, one bite at a time.*

Val's Pickled Cauliflower

⅓ cup white balsamic vinegar

⅓ cup rice wine vinegar

⅓ cup apple cider vinegar

1½ cups water

1 tablespoon salt

2 cloves of garlic

2 bay leaves

1 teaspoon mustard seeds

2 chiles de arbol (fresh or dry)

1 small cauliflower head, cut into florets

Combine all ingredients except the cauliflower in a small pot and bring to a boil. Stir in the cauliflower and then remove from heat. Let cool to room temperature.

Once cool, distribute cauliflower evenly between two 32-ounce glass jars with one garlic clove, bay leaf and chile in each jar. Cover with the liquid and refrigerate. The pickled cauliflower will last about two months. Be sure to use a clean fork to remove florets from the jar to make them last longer.

In the summer months this recipe can be used for cucumber and zucchini.

Austin's Guacamole

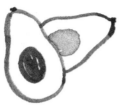

Austin Spivey is the Business Operations Manager at Zoomer, a San Francisco-based company that provides outsourced delivery for high-volume restaurants. Born in Illinois, Austin lived and worked in the fashion industry in New York City for six years before moving to the land of avocados.

Austin's Guacamole

3 tablespoons minced and drained roma or grape tomatoes

2 tablespoons minced yellow onion

2 tablespoons minced jalapeño pepper

2 tablespoons minced fresh cilantro

½ teaspoon salt

3-4 avocados, skin and pit removed, chopped

1 teaspoon fresh lime juice

Stir together tomato, onion, jalapeño, cilantro and salt. Add avocado and lime juice and mix well. The avocado will get slightly mashed but still have some chunks. Serve immediately or seal tightly with plastic wrap to store in refrigerator for up to 2 hours.

Vincent's Nachos

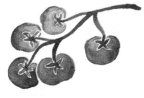

Vincent Lesage is an art lover and the inspired executive chef at Bacara Resort & Spa in Santa Barbara, California. Born and raised in Paris, Vincent graduated from Institut Paul Bocuse before training at The Ritz Paris, followed by the Michelin three-star restaurants L'Astrance and Bras. His love of art continues to influence his artistic food presentation.

Vincent's Nachos
serves 6 as appetizer

2 taro roots or 1 sweet potato, peeled and sliced into thin "chips"

1 avocado, diced

1 bunch green onions, sliced fresh cilantro leaves for garnish

For Cashew Cream
2 cups raw cashew nuts

2 cups water

1 jalapeño, seeded and sliced

1 teaspoon minced garlic

salt to taste

For Pickled Tomato
1 pound whole heirloom cherry tomatoes

2 teaspoons olive oil

1 teaspoon balsamic vinegar

1 clove garlic, minced

½ bunch cilantro, minced

Prepare the cashew cream and pickled tomato.

For cashew cream, soak the cashews in warm water for an hour with the jalapeño and garlic. Blend everything in mixer until smooth. Add salt to taste.

For pickled tomato, heat the olive oil in a pan over medium heat until it starts to smoke. Add cherry tomatoes and cook until they start to blister. Remove from heat, add the garlic and vinegar. Set aside to marinate for an hour. Stir in cilantro when ready to serve.

For chips, spread taro root slices in a single layer on a foil-lined baking sheet. Bake in a preheated oven at 280°F for 15 minutes until crispy.

In a bowl, assemble 2 or 3 layers, starting each layer with taro root, adding cashew cream, pickled tomato, green onion slices and avocado chunks. Top with cilantro.

Evey's Dip & Chips

Evey Schweig, AADP, is a certified Holistic Health Coach with degrees in biology and integrated nutrition. She works with clients as a personal guide to help them achieve more energy-filled, pain-free lives and is a staunch advocate of eating nutritious whole foods to improve health and maintain optimal weight. She publishes a blog and newsletter on healthy eating and lifestyle at www.eveyschweig.com. Evey lives in Glencoe, Illinois, with her husband and two children.

Evey's Dip and Chips
serves a crowd

For Dip
2 sweet potatoes (about 1½ pounds), peeled and cut into ½-inch cubes

2 tablespoons olive oil, divided

1½ teaspoons cumin

¼ teaspoon turmeric

¼ teaspoon salt

⅛ teaspoon pepper

⅓ cup tahini

¼ cup fresh-squeezed lemon juice

1 clove garlic, minced

4-6 tablespoons water

salt and pepper to taste

paprika for garnish

Preheat oven to 400°F.

In a bowl, combine sweet potatoes with 1 tablespoon olive oil, cumin, turmeric, salt and pepper. Mix until evenly coated. Place into 9-x-13-inch roasting pan. Loosely cover and bake 25 minutes. Stir and bake uncovered for an additional 20 minutes or until the potatoes are very soft. Remove from oven and let cool.

Place cooled sweet potatoes into food processor. Add garlic and pulse until smooth. Add remaining 1 tablespoon of olive oil, tahini, and lemon juice. Pulse until well blended. Slowly add water until a smooth, creamy consistency is reached. Season with additional salt and pepper if desired.

Garnish with a drizzle of olive oil and a sprinkle of paprika. Enjoy with crudités or Evey's grain-free chips.

For Chips
makes 2 dozen

1 ripe banana

⅜ cup (6 tablespoons) golden flaxseeds

2 tablespoons ground flax

1 tablespoon black sesame seeds

¼ teaspoon cinnamon

¼ teaspoon salt

2-3 tablespoons water

Preheat oven to 300°F. Line two baking sheets with parchment paper.

In a medium bowl, mash banana with a fork until smooth. Add all other ingredients except water, and hand mix until well incorporated. Let sit for 10 minutes or more to allow the batter to thicken. If batter becomes too thick to easily scoop, add water to thin it.

Using a teaspoon, drop small mounds of batter about 2 inches apart on baking sheets. Using the bottom of a wet measuring cup, flatten mounds to about ⅛-inch thickness. Thinner is better, as you will get a crispier chip.

Bake for 20 minutes. Flip each chip with a spatula and return to oven for 20-30 minutes more. You may want to rearrange the outer chips to the middle to ensure even cooking. They are done when lightly browned and crisp.

Remove from oven and cool on wire racks. Store refrigerated in an airtight container for several days. If crackers get soggy, crisp them up in a 300°F oven for 10-15 minutes.

Sanford's Shishitos

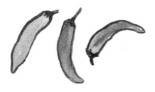

Sanford Spivey is a Business Development Analyst at Sonos, the company that is reinventing home audio for the digital age with wireless speakers. Sanford began his career at Sonos while playing on the Boston University Men's Soccer Team and getting his degree in Entrepreneurship from BU's Questrom School of Business. He was born in Mexico City, Mexico, which may be why he loves peppers.

Sanford's Shishitos

8 ounces fresh shishito peppers

2 teaspoons olive oil

¼ teaspoon salt

Heat olive oil in large pan over medium-high heat and add peppers. Toss peppers in pan for 6-8 minutes or until blistering and turning soft. Sprinkle with salt and serve.

Sheridan's Plantains

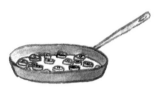

Sheridan Spivey took a leave of absence from Duke University to work as Event Operations Senior Associate for the Bay Area Super Bowl 50 Host Committee. In August 2016, Sheridan returns to Duke to complete her senior year. Born in Melbourne, Australia, Sheridan understands there is a difference between Aussie rules and gridiron football.

Sheridan's Plantains

2-3 yellow or partially black plantains

2 tablespoons olive oil

¼ teaspoon salt

Peel and slice plantains into ¼-inch coins. Heat olive oil in a large pan over medium heat. Add plantains in a single layer (in batches if necessary) and cook without stirring 3-5 minutes or until browned on one side. Flip and cook another few minutes until the plantains are nicely browned and soft but not mushy. Sprinkle with salt and serve.

Maureen's Househ & Eggs

Maureen Abood is a chef, writer, photographer and the author of the critically acclaimed cookbook Rose Water & Orange Blossoms: Fresh and Classic Recipes from My Lebanese Kitchen *(Running Press 2015), listed in Publishers Weekly "Top 10 Cookbooks" in Spring 2015. Her award-winning blog of the same name chronicles her recipes, life in Northern Michigan, and stories about growing up in a Lebanese-American kitchen. Maureen's family makes Lebanese househ and eggs for breakfast when they want a protein-rich, strong and delicious start to the day.*

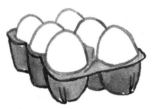

Maureen's Househ & Eggs
serves 4–6

2 tablespoons olive oil

½ yellow onion, finely diced (½ cup)

½ pound grass-fed ground beef

¼ teaspoon cinnamon

½ teaspoon salt or to taste

¼ teaspoon pepper or to taste

juice of ½ lemon (2 tablespoons)

2 tablespoons toasted pine nuts

10 eggs, lightly beaten

10 grape tomatoes, halved, for garnish

In a medium pan, heat the olive oil over medium heat until hot but not smoking. Add the onion and cook until soft and translucent. (Do not brown.) Add the beef and stir, breaking the meat into small pieces as it browns, until the meat is cooked through. Add cinnamon, salt, pepper, and lemon juice. Stir in the pine nuts.

Still over medium heat, pour eggs over the meat and gently nudge the eggs as curds form. Cook until the eggs are soft-scrambled with the meat. Serve immediately, garnished with tomatoes.

Tanya's ABC Soup

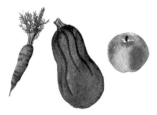

Tanya Steel is an award-winning cookbook author who was Editor-in-Chief of Epicurious, Editor-in-Chief of Gourmet Live and Gourmet. com, and an Editor at Bon Appetit and Food and Wine, in addition to writing for numerous other publications including the New York Times and Travel & Leisure. She conceived of The Kids State Dinner, is Award Director of the Julia Child Award and runs her own multimedia culinary agency.

Tanya's ABC Soup (Apple, Butternut Squash & Carrots)
serves 6–8

1 medium butternut squash (2 pounds) peeled, seeded, and quartered

½ teaspoon nutmeg

2 medium Granny Smith apples, peeled, cored and quartered

1 tablespoon melted coconut oil, plus extra for greasing pan

2-3 carrots, peeled and chopped (1 generous cup)

1 medium onion, peeled and chopped (1 generous cup)

2 garlic cloves, peeled and minced

¼ teaspoon turmeric

2 cups chicken stock

1-2 cups water

Preheat oven to 350°F. Line a baking pan with foil and grease the foil with ½ teaspoon melted coconut oil. Place squash quarters onto the foil and sprinkle with nutmeg. Bake 20 minutes. Add apples and cook 20 minutes more, or until squash and apples are soft when pierced with a knife. Let cool.

In a large pan, warm coconut oil and add carrots and onion. Cook over low heat, stirring occasionally, for 5-7 minutes. Add garlic and turmeric and cook 5-7 minutes more, or until softened but not browned. Let cool.

Put squash, apples, carrots, and onion mixture in a blender with the chicken stock and puree until smooth. Add water, ½ cup at a time, and blend until reaching desired consistency. Refrigerate until serving.

In a large pot over medium-low heat, reheat soup gently and serve warm.

Jane's Eggs Benedict

Jane Biscarini fell in love with Italy, and its food culture during college, then married an Italian and lived there full-time for 14 years, learning the secrets of Italian cooking from her family and friends and teaching at the US Embassy in Rome. Jane now lives and teaches cooking half of each year in Chattanooga, Tennessee, where she runs the tour company eatsipwalk.com with her family.

Jane's Eggs Benedict
serves 2–4

1 acorn squash

½ teaspoon salt

4 tablespoons olive oil, separated

4 eggs

8 ounces baby spinach

4 ounces prosciutto, thin sliced

½ avocado, peeled and sliced

cracked black pepper to serve

For Hollandaise
½ cup melted ghee

1 tablespoon fresh lemon juice

2 egg yolks

Preheat oven to 400° F.

Cut squash in half and remove seeds. Slice off four ½-inch rings and coat with 2 tablespoons of the olive oil. (Reserve remaining squash for another use.) Place rings on parchment-lined sheet pan, sprinkle with salt and roast 25 minutes or until fork tender.

While squash is roasting, make hollandaise. When squash is done, remove from oven and begin cooking eggs.

In a large skillet, warm the remaining 2 tablespoons of olive oil over medium-low heat and crack in eggs. Cover the pan and watch carefully about 4 minutes or until each egg white is firm and yolk still soft. During the last minute of cooking the eggs, add all the spinach to the pan and cover to wilt the spinach while beginning to assemble plates.

Place 1 or 2 slices of roasted squash on a plate, top each squash with a slice of prosciutto, then spinach, 1 egg, and slices of avocado. Drizzle hollandaise sauce over and top with ground pepper.

For hollandaise, whisk 2 egg yolks with the lemon juice for 2 minutes or until pale and thickened. Add the melted ghee 1 drop at a time and continue whisking until emulsified and thick. It's very important to add the ghee very slowly or the sauce does not emulsify.

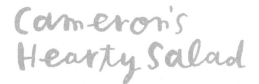

Cameron's Hearty Salad

Cameron Silver is the Fashion Director of H By Halston and a premier QVC personality. He is the founder of vintage clothing empire Decades *and best-selling author of* Decades: A Century of Fashion. *As the star of the popular Bravo series* Dukes of Melrose, *Cameron was aptly named King of Vintage. A Los Angeles native, Cameron is currently based in New York City.*

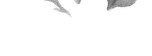

Cameron's Hearty Salad
serves 4

For Dressing
1 tablespoon cold-pressed walnut oil (optional but good for flavor depth)

⅔ cup minus 1 tablespoon cold-pressed olive oil (mix brands for best flavor)

⅓ cup fresh lemon juice

1 teaspoon balsamic vinegar

1 tablespoon French grain mustard

¼ teaspoon pressed garlic cloves

½ teaspoon salt or to taste

¼ teaspoon pepper or to taste

For Salad
4 cups organic salad greens

2 carrots, diced

1 heirloom tomato, chopped (or substitute diced roasted beets in winter)

¼ cup pitted olives, chopped

1 6.7-oz jar Tonnino tuna fillets in olive oil

1-2 hard boiled eggs (optional)

1 avocado, sliced (optional)

For dressing, whisk together all ingredients. Can be kept in the refrigerator for a week.

For salad, toss all ingredients except tuna, eggs, and avocado in a large bowl with ¼ cup dressing. Separate onto 4 serving plates. Divide tuna, egg and avocado evenly among the plates. Drizzle more dressing over top if desired.

Maili's Tomato Ginger Salmon

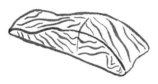

Maili Halme has a passion for food and cooking. She is a professional chef and caterer with a long list of celebrity clients. Maili documents many of her stories and recipes on her blog and webpage www. mailihalme.com. She is based in Solvang, California, where her mother and sister founded The Solvang Bakery.

Maili's Tomato Ginger Salmon
serves 6

For Sauce
3 tablespoons olive oil

3 tablespoons minced ginger

2 teaspoons minced garlic

3 cups grape or cherry tomatoes sliced in halves

1 tablespoon honey

½ teaspoon salt or to taste

pinch of red pepper flakes

For Salmon
6 servings of salmon (4 ounces each)

¼ cup cold-pressed olive oil

2 teaspoons salt

fresh basil leaves for garnish

For sauce, pour olive oil in a sauté pan over medium heat. Add ginger and garlic and sauté about 1 minute. Be careful not to burn! Add tomatoes, honey, salt and red pepper flakes. Stir to combine and cook about 5-7 minutes or until liquid is almost evaporated and tomatoes are soft. Remove from heat.

For salmon, place a clean and dry pan over high heat. Coat the salmon pieces with oil and sprinkle with salt. Place salmon in hot pan and leave for 2-4 minutes until a brown crust is formed. Flip over and cook another few minutes until fish is not quite cooked through. Set salmon on plate and spoon warm sauce over top. Garnish with basil.

Kathleen Cochran is Goleta's 2015 Woman of the Year and a 35-year veteran of the luxury hospitality industry. She is the Vice President Operations and Managing Director of The Resort at Paw's Up, in western Montana. Her career includes posts at the Bacara Resort & Spa, Plaza Hotel, Hotel del Coronado and Loews Hotels. She received numerous accolades for her management success, industry innovations and community collaborations. Kathleen is an avid cook and rose gardener who puts cookbooks at the top of her reading list.

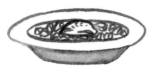

Kathleen's Turkey Hash with Eggs

serves 4

2 tablespoons ghee or clarified butter

1 cup diced onion

1 red chile, finely minced

1 cup diced red bell pepper

½ teaspoon kosher salt to taste

1 pinch nutmeg

1 pinch cayenne pepper

2-4 cloves garlic, minced

2 cups diced, cooked turkey breast

1 cup diced, cooked acorn squash

2 teaspoons minced chives

2 teaspoons minced fresh cilantro

8 large eggs

2 cups chicken broth

1 teaspoon fresh lemon juice

Cranberry Relish (optional)
4 ounces fresh cranberries

2 teaspoons maple syrup

2 teaspoons honey

½ medium orange, zested and juiced

1 tablespoon minced mint

Melt butter in large pan over medium heat and add onions, chili, pepper, salt, nutmeg and cayenne. Cook 3-5 minutes or until just starting to brown. Turn heat to medium low and add garlic. Cook 1 minute and stir in turkey. Gently add squash and ½ the chives and cilantro. Heat through.

Simultaneously, poach the eggs in simmering chicken stock with squeeze of lemon in broth.

Divide hash onto 4 plates and make a crater in the center of each for eggs. Place two poached eggs in each crater and sprinkle with remaining herbs. Place a spoonful of cranberry relish in a line over the eggs and serve.

For relish, pulse all ingredients in a food processor until reaching desired consistency. Relish should be in small chunks, not pureed. Allow to rest and mature at least 30 minutes. Serve chilled or at room temperature.

Lynda's Roast Veggies & Chicken

Lynda Weinman is an author, speaker, teacher, animator, and the co-founder of lynda.com, which was sold to LinkedIn in the fourth largest deal in social media history. Lynda is a self-trained digital media and graphics expert who authored Designing Web Graphics, *the first book about web technologies from a visual-design perspective.*

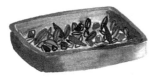

Lynda's Roast Veggies & Chicken
serves 4

⅓ cup olive oil

2 cloves garlic, finely minced

2 teaspoons dried rosemary

2 teaspoons plus ¼ teaspoon salt

¼ teaspoon pepper

8-10 cups vegetables cut into bite-sized pieces (cauliflower, butternut squash, brussels sprouts or whatever is in season)

1½ pounds organic chicken thighs, cut into bite-sized pieces

2 teaspoons balsamic vinegar

1 tablespoon hot sauce (optional)

Preheat oven to 400°F. Whisk together oil, garlic, rosemary, 2 teaspoons salt and the pepper in a large bowl. Add vegetables and toss well. Turn out onto a large (12-x-18-inch) rimmed baking sheet or pan. Put chicken pieces in same bowl and toss with vinegar and ¼ teaspoon salt. Place chicken pieces in one layer on top of vegetables.

Roast for 20 minutes. Remove from oven and toss together using 2 large spoons. Turn oven to 350°F and cook another 20 minutes or until cooked through. Serve in bowls with a drizzle of your favorite hot sauce, if desired.

Marni's Stir-Fry

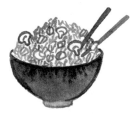

Marni Blau Margerum writes her lifestyle blog, Wine is Good Living *as a way to combine her passion for food and travel with her background in fashion and interior design, and wine as the omnipresent theme in her daily life (which she shares with husband Doug Margerum, owner and winemaker of Margerum Wine Company.) Marni's blog depicts her personal style of entertaining and design, and she offers hand-curated treasures both online and in Margerum's Santa Barbara tasting room.*

Marni's Stir Fry
serves 3–4

1 head of cauliflower, cut into florets

2 tablespoons olive oil, separated

1 teaspoon chile oil

1 small yellow onion, chopped (1 cup)

2 cups broccoli florets

½ red bell pepper, stemmed, seeded and sliced

2 cups sliced mushrooms

1 teaspoon minced garlic

¼ cup chicken stock

¼ cup coconut aminos

1 tablespoon grated fresh ginger

¾ pound pork loin, chopped into bite-sized pieces (can be substituted with any animal protein)

Pulse the cauliflower florets in a food processor until finely chopped and resembling rice.

Heat 1 tablespoon olive oil and the chile oil in wok (or large skillet) over medium heat. Add onions and cook for about 5-6 minutes. Add broccoli, pepper and mushrooms. Stir for 2 minutes and add garlic, chicken stock and cauliflower. Cook another 5-7 minutes or until vegetables are tender, then stir in coconut aminos and ginger. Remove from heat.

Add remaining 1 tablespoon olive oil to a separate skillet over medium heat and cook pork 5-7 minutes. Add the pork to the vegetables and stir until pork is cooked through. Serve hot.

Karen's Crab Cakes (with mango salsa)

Karen Sipprell managed some of the original marketing communications teams at Apple that launched the iPhone, iPad, iPod and Macintosh. She currently teaches company culture and management philosophy at Apple University and consults to Apple's global business leaders regarding learning and development initiatives for their teams. Karen loves to make crab cakes for her husband and son.

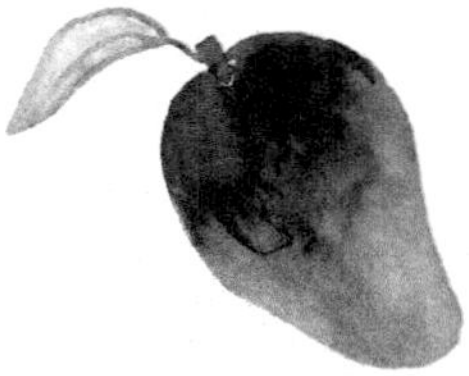

Karen's Crab Cakes (with mango salsa)

serves 6–8

For Crab Cakes

½ pound cooked bay shrimp

½ pound fresh crabmeat

3 tablespoons finely diced celery

1 tablespoon finely diced shallot

1 tablespoon minced fresh dill

1 tablespoon minced chives

1 tablespoon Dijon mustard

2 teaspoons lemon zest

½ teaspoon paprika

¼ teaspoon cayenne

¼ teaspoon black pepper

2 egg yolks

4 tablespoons melted ghee, separated

For Salsa

1 mango, diced (2 cups)

2 tablespoons diced red onion

2 tablespoons peeled and diced cucumber

1 tablespoon chopped cilantro leaves

2 tablespoons fresh lime juice

½ teaspoon honey

¼ teaspoon of salt

For salsa, mix all ingredients together and refrigerate 1 hour before serving.

For crab cakes, pulse shrimp in a food processor until just chopped. Add crab and pulse just to incorporate. You still want pieces of shrimp and crab evident. Turn out onto paper towel and pat dry.

In a medium bowl, combine celery, shallot, dill and chives. Stir in mustard, lemon zest, paprika and peppers. Add shrimp and crab and mix until combined. Stir in egg yolks and 2 tablespoons of melted ghee.

Roll 2-inch balls of seafood mixture and flatten to ½-inch-thick patties onto a baking sheet or plate. Refrigerate for one hour.

In a pan over medium high heat, melt 2 remaining tablespoons ghee and cook crab cakes for 3 minutes on each side. Turn off heat and let sit in pan for 2-5 minutes.

Serve hot with cold mango salsa.

Ray's Sausages & Peppers

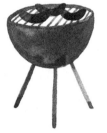

Ray Landy is the former President and CEO of AECOM Architecture, one of the largest global architecture and engineering firms, overseeing such prestigious projects as the Louvre and Guggenheim museums in Abu Dhabi and terminals at both SFO and JFK airports. Ray's affinity for peppers began in his youth in Texas and developed while he was living in Tunisia and Morocco while in the Peace Corps. He now grows his own peppers and focuses on his current passion of painting.

Ray's Sausages & Peppers
serves 4

4 tablespoons apple cider vinegar

2 tablespoons olive oil

½ teaspoon kosher salt or to taste

¼ teaspoon ground pepper or to taste

1 large onion cut into 1-inch pieces

2 cups sweet and/or bell peppers cut into 2-inch long slices

2 tablespoons hot peppers (jalapeño or serrano) cut into ¼-inch pieces

2 pounds fresh chicken sausage with no added fillers

2-3 tablespoons whole grain Dijon mustard

Combine vinegar, oil, salt and pepper in a large container and add onion, peppers and sausages. Mix and refrigerate, covered, for several hours.

Heat a grill basket on a barbeque or a large skillet on the stove. Add the onion, peppers and sausages and cook over high heat for about 10 minutes or until vegetables are charred but still crisp. Remove from heat and move sausages to the barbeque grill or a grill pan and sear or brown until cooked through. Remove sausages, cut into 1-inch slices and toss well in a bowl with the mustard. Serve sausages on top of the grilled vegetables with extra mustard on the side.

Frances' Beef Curry

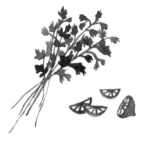

Frances Schultz is a journalist, tastemaker, world traveler, hostess, Southerner, Sunday painter and outdoors lover. She is author and co-author of several books, including Atlanta at Table *and* The Bee Cottage Story—How I Made a Muddle of Things and Decorated My Way Back to Happiness. *Frances is also a contributing editor to* House Beautiful *magazine, former editor-at-large for* Veranda, *and was on-air host of* Southern Living Presents.

Frances' Beef Curry
serves 4

4 ounces red curry paste

2 cups coconut milk

1 pound flank steak or London broil, cut into ¼-inch slices

fresh cilantro and limes to garnish

In a large pot over medium heat, cook curry paste for 2 minutes. Turn heat to low, stir in coconut milk and add beef slices. Cover and cook 1½ to 2 hours or until beef is tender.

Serve over vegetables or zucchini noodles and garnish with a spring of cilantro and a wedge of fresh lime, if desired.

Ronnie's Meatloaf

Ronnie Lott is one of the greatest defensive backs in football history and has been inducted into both the College and Pro Football Hall of Fame. He played in four winning Super Bowls for the San Francisco 49ers and played for the Oakland Raiders and New York Jets in subsequent years. In 2015, Ronnie was honored as the Pac 12 Defensive Player of the Century. He spends his time now working in support of his charity, All Stars Helping Kids, which has raised over $20 million for underserved youth. He enjoys his favorite meatloaf at Nick's Next Door in Los Gatos, California.

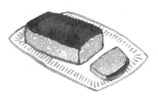

Ronnie's Meatloaf (with sweet and spicy sauce)

serves 6

For Meatloaf

2-3 chopped carrots (1 cup)

1 chopped yellow onion (1 cup)

3 cups chopped button mushrooms (6-8 ounces)

1 pound grass-fed ground beef

1 pound ground pork

1 egg

3 tablespoons tomato paste

¼ cup dry Italian seasoning

1 teaspoon salt

¼ teaspoon pepper

1 teaspoon olive oil for greasing pan

For Sauce (optional)

1 teaspoon minced garlic

1 teaspoon minced ginger

2 teaspoons finely chopped scallion

1 tablespoon honey

1 tablespoon chile paste (sambal oelek)*

½ cup hoisin*

*Chili paste and hoisin can contain ingredients that are not Paleo. Recipes to make Paleo versions of these condiments are readily available online.

Preheat oven to 375°F on convection or 400°F regular bake.

For meatloaf, puree carrots, onions and mushrooms in a food processor. Cook mixture on the stove in a pan over medium heat about 10–15 minutes, until moisture has evaporated and mixture is very dry. Remove from heat and cool 15 minutes.

Mix together pork and beef in a large bowl and stir in egg, tomato paste, Italian seasoning, salt and pepper. Add vegetable puree and mix together well with gloved hands, patting down to remove air bubbles.

Grease a 5-x-9-inch loaf pan with olive oil and fill with meat mixture. Cook about 30 minutes (or 40 minutes on non-convection) until meat registers 135°F in the center. (It should be pink, so it can cook through at second cooking.) Cool down and refrigerate several hours or overnight.

Slice in 1¼-inch pieces and place on foil-lined baking sheet. Cook in preheated 350°F oven until hot in the center, about 20 minutes. Serve with sauce drizzled on top if desired.

For sauce, whisk all ingredients together in a bowl. Refrigerate until ready to use. Warm gently before serving.

Barry's Beef Stew

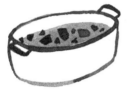

Barry Johnson has always been a foodie, but for the past six years he has been a Paleo foodie and loves to use his pressure cooker to create fast and fresh dinners. Barry is a renowned interior and furniture designer, known for his color sense and unique custom furniture. He shares his design talents, and his food, with the innovators of Silicon Valley, where he lives and works.

Barry's Beef Stew
serves 4

2 tablespoons olive oil

1½ pounds lean beef, cut into cubes

3 cloves garlic, chopped

1 large celery root bulb, peeled and cut into 1-inch cubes

1 yellow onion, chopped (2 cups)

1 red bell pepper, cored and chopped

2-3 carrots, chopped (1 cup)

2-3 stalks celery, chopped (3/4 cup)

2 tablespoons Herbes de Provence

1 teaspoon salt

¼ teaspoon black pepper

1 tablespoon Sriracha hot chili sauce (optional)*

fresh Italian parsley leaves for garnish

*Sriracha may contain ingredients that are not Paleo. Recipes are available online to make Paleo Sriracha if you desire.

Heat olive oil in a frying pan over high heat. Add beef and sear the meat, stirring to brown on all sides. Remove from heat and stir in garlic, being careful not to burn the garlic. Put the beef and garlic with any remaining olive oil into a Crock Pot or pressure cooker.

Add 2 cups of water to the pot, then add celery root, onions, red bell pepper, carrots, celery, herbs, salt, pepper and Sriracha, if desired.

Cook in a Crock Pot on high for 5 hours or until vegetables are tender and stew is fragrant. Or secure the lid of the pressure cooker and heat on the stove until the needle of the pressure cooker goes to its highest, then reduce the heat until the needle rests midpoint. Continue cooking at midpoint level for 20 minutes, then turn off heat and let rest for 15 minutes before releasing the lid.

Ladle the stew into bowls and top with chopped fresh Italian parsley.

Leslie's Ginger Cookies

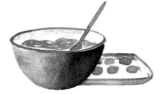

Leslie McFadden is a real estate agent with Village Properties, an affiliate of Christie's International Real Estate. Leslie joined the real estate world after working in design for over a decade, collaborating on interiors and architecture for both commercial and residential renovation projects throughout Southern California. Leslie appreciates the Santa Barbara lifestyle, fostering lasting relationships and connecting old and new friends.

Leslie's Ginger Cookies
makes 2 dozen

3 cups finely ground almond flour

½ teaspoon salt

½ teaspoon baking soda

2 teaspoons ground ginger

1 teaspoon ground cinnamon

½ teaspoon ground cloves

¼ cup melted coconut oil

¼ cup melted butter or ghee

⅓ cup molasses

3 tablespoons honey

1 teaspoon grated fresh ginger

Preheat oven to 350°F.

Mix flour, salt, baking soda, ground ginger, cinnamon and cloves in food processor and pulse to blend.

Stir oil, butter or ghee, molasses and grated ginger together and add to food processor. Mix until well blended. The batter will be greasy.

Roll dough into walnut-sized balls and gently press onto a baking sheet lined with parchment paper.

Bake 10-13 minutes until slight cracks appear on top.

Leela's Fig Flan

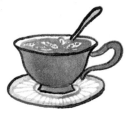

Leela Cyd is a photographer and author living in Santa Barbara, California. She shoots for a range of publications including The New York Times, Kinfolk, *and* Sweet Paul Magazine. *Her commercial work centers around artisan food, design and lifestyle. Leela's cookbook,* Food with Friends, *was published in March 2016.*

Leela's Fig Flan
serves 5

3 tablespoons melted ghee

3 tablespoons honey

3 eggs

¼ cup almond meal

1 large pinch salt

1 vanilla bean, split and scraped

¾ cup coconut milk

1 pint fresh figs, cut into quarters

2 tablespoons slivered almonds

2 tablespoons unsweetened coconut flakes

Preheat oven to 400°F. Melt ghee in microwave or in a pot on low. Brush 5 heat-proof teacups with melted ghee and set aside, reserving any ghee that wasn't used in this process.

In a medium bowl, whisk honey, eggs, almond meal, salt, contents of the vanilla bean (vanilla pod can be discarded) and coconut milk together until incorporated. Divide figs evenly among the 5 teacups and pour egg mixture over the figs. Drizzle any remaining ghee over the top. Place the teacups on a pan and bake for about 10 minutes.

Remove from oven, sprinkle almonds and coconut onto the semi-set flans, and return to oven for another 10-15 minutes, until tops are golden brown. Remove from oven. The flans are best served warm but are fine after a few hours at room temperature.

Elizabeth's Coconut Macaroons

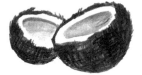

Elizabeth Colling is an acclaimed pastry chef and proprietor of Merci To Go, an organic homemade food store in Montecito, California. She earned her degree at the Ritz Escoffier in Paris before working at Spago Beverly Hills and becoming the pastry chef at Bastide. Elizabeth was a Food Editor for Martha Stewart Living *and* Martha Stewart Weddings *magazines, where she developed and styled desserts for both publications.*

Elizabeth's Coconut Macaroons (dipped in chocolate)
makes about 10

For Macaroons
1 teaspoon melted coconut oil

3 egg whites

½ vanilla bean, split and scraped

¼ teaspoon vanilla extract

¼ teaspoon kosher salt

¼ cup honey

1¾ cups unsweetened shredded coconut

For Chocolate
¼ cup coconut oil

2 tablespoons honey

¼ teaspoon kosher salt

½ cup unsweetened cocoa powder

Preheat oven to 325°F. Line a baking pan with parchment paper and then grease paper with the coconut oil.

For macaroons, whisk together the egg whites, contents of the vanilla bean (vanilla pod can be discarded), vanilla extract and salt in a medium metal bowl set over a pot of simmering water. Add the honey and whisk intermittently until very warm to the touch, about 2-3 minutes. The mixture should look frothy. Remove from heat.

Add the coconut and fold into the warm mixture until all of the liquid is absorbed. You may need to let it sit for a few minutes and fold again.

Fill a 1-ounce mini ice cream scoop (1¾-inch diameter) with batter and pack to make a compact scoop. Place each scoop 1 inch apart on pan and bake for 25 minutes or until the macaroons are a deep golden brown. Let cool completely before dipping in chocolate.

For chocolate, combine the coconut oil, honey and salt in a small pot. Heat to melt the coconut oil. Place the cocoa powder in a small bowl and pour the warm mixture over cocoa powder. Whisk to combine.

Dip the cooled macaroons into the chocolate, coating the bottom of the macaroon (and up about a quarter of the macaroon or as far as you desire.) Place each on a parchment-lined cookie sheet and refrigerate to set.

Macaroons are best the day they are baked but can be stored refrigerated in an airtight container for up to 2 days.

Jenni's Almond Cake

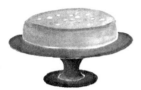

Jenni Kayne is an American designer best known for her timeless wardrobe classics. Through Rip & Tan, her lifestyle blog named after her children, she seamlessly weaves together stories and images of modern family tradition with sublime design taste. Jenni's inviting minimalist aesthetic translates effortlessly from her apparel collection to home, entertaining, travel and food.

Jenni's Almond Cake

1½ cups almond meal

1 teaspoon baking power*

8 egg whites

½ cup maple syrup

1 teaspoon vanilla extract

zest of 2 oranges
(2 tablespoons)

½ cup melted coconut oil
plus extra for greasing pan

1 teaspoon cinnamon

1 teaspoon coconut
palm sugar

1 cup sliced almonds

fresh berries for serving

*Baking powder can contain non-Paleo ingredients. If desired, make your own with 1 teaspoon baking soda mixed with 2 teaspoons cream of tartar.

Preheat oven to 350° F. Combine almond meal and baking powder in a small bowl. In a large bowl, whisk the egg whites until they are foamy and start to hold their shape. Slowly add the maple syrup, whisking until the mixture is thick and shiny. Add the vanilla extract and the orange zest.

Alternately whisk in the coconut oil with almond meal and baking powder in thirds until they are smoothly incorporated into the egg whites. Pour the mixture into a 9-inch spring-form pan that has been greased with coconut oil.

Mix together cinnamon and sugar. Sprinkle ½ the mixture on top of the batter, then sprinkle on all the almonds. Sprinkle the remaining cinnamon and sugar on top.

Bake for 30-40 minutes, or until the top has risen and set, the almonds become golden and a cake tester comes out clean.

Remove the cake from the oven and let it cool completely. Once cool, remove from pan. Serve with berries.

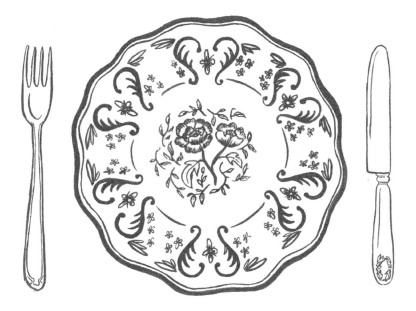

and so on
and so forth...

THANK YOU

MAUREEN ABOOD · Mikaila Allison
Pascale Beale · Jane Biscarini
THE BLACKWELL FAMILY
BARET BOISSON · Merryl Brown
Kathy Burt · KATHLEEN COCHRAN
Janey Cohen · Elizabeth Colling
Kendall Conrad · MARYANNE
CONTRERAS · Leela Cyd
Suzy Davidson · LINDA DITTMANN
Jim Dodge · ANNE ELCON · Winn Ellis
ROBIN FELL · The Flick Family · Jessica Foster
Barb Galiotto · JODI GOLDBERG
JOHN GRAY · Beth Green · MOLLY
GREEN · JESSE GROVES · Lisa
Hagerman · MAILI HALME · Victoria
Harvey · BRUCE HEAVIN
Carolyn Hill · Tammy Hughes · Mac Irvin
Chana Jackson · HOLLYE JACOBS
Barry Johnson · LAURA MACKER JOHNSTON
Jenni Kayne · Dawn Lafitte

RAY LANDY · Kate Lepp · VINCENT LESAGE · KAREN & RONNIE LOTT · PATTY MACFARLANE · Doug Margerum · Marni Blau Margerum · Melissa Marsted Alixe Mattingly · SUSAN MCCAW · SHEILA MCCONVILLE Leslie McFadden · Anne Milling · JILLIAN MULLER · Melodee Myers · MATT PESENDIAN · Debby Peterson Lizzy Deus · MARLA PHILLIPS SUSAN PITCHER · Robin Poett JENNIFER POWELL · Elizabeth Raith · Valerie Rice · KELLY SAMUELS · Jo Saxon · Frances Schultz · EVEY SCHWEIG · Laura Shelburne · STEPHANIE SHIRO Sue Siegel · Cameron Silver · Karen Sipprell · THE SPIVEY FAMILY · TANYA STEEL · Daryl Stegall · The Thomas Family · Rebecca Votto LYNDA WEINMAN · Kimberly Wilcox

LET FOOD BE THY MEDICINE and MEDICINE BE THY FOOD.

HIPPOCRATES

GOING BEYOND

This book was written to provide you with basic information about being Paleo and perhaps inspire you to learn more. You will find, as I did, that writers vary in their Paleo information. It is important to determine what works specifically for you and your life.

This list of websites will help you continue your Paleo journey. While it is by no means a comprehensive list, from these sites you can learn about additional resources, including books, blogs, podcasts, apps, conferences, foods and services. There are hundreds, if not thousands of Paleo resources, so enjoy the learning!

Alderspring Ranch | alderspring.com

Amy Densmore | paleocupboard.com

Arsy Vartanian | rubiesandradishes.com

Barefoot Provisions | barefootprovisions.com

Chris Kresser | chriskresser.com

Danielle Walker | againstallgrain.com

Diane Sanfilippo | balancedbites.com

Dr. Kellyann Petrucci | drkellyann.com

Kelly Brozyna | thespunkycoconut.com

Liz Wolfe | realfoodliz.com

Loren Cordain | thepaleodiet.com

Mark Sisson | marksdailyapple.com

Melissa and Dallas Hartwig | whole9life.com

Melissa Joulwan | meljoulwan.com

Michelle Tam | nomnompaleo.com

Paleohacks | blog.paleohacks.com/about/

Paleo Leap | paleoleap.com

Paleo Magazine | paleomagonline.com

Paleo Plan | paleoplan.com

Pete Evans | peteevans.com

Primal Palate | primalpalate.com

Primal Pastures | primalpastures.com

Robb Wolf | robbwolf.com

Sarah Ballantyne, PhD | thepaleomom.com

Sarah Fragoso | sarahfragoso.com

Sweet Laurel | sweetlaurel.com

Terry Wahls, M.D. | terrywahls.com

Thrive Market | thrivemarket.com

U.S. Wellness Meats | grasslandbeef.com

Vital Choice | vitalchoice.com/shop/pc/newsletter-signup.asp

INDEX

green beans, 29, 35
green drink/green juice, 57
Guacamole, 102
gut health, 29, 32, 38, 61, 92

H
Halme, Maili, 99, 113
Hartwig, Melissa and Dallas, 137
heart, 26, 60
heart disease, 57
Hearty Salad, 112
herbs, 94
history of Paleo, 7-11
hoisin, 122
hollandaise, 110-111
homo erectus, 9
homo sapiens, 9.11
honey, 25, 34, 38, 41, 94
hormones, 38, 57, 69
hot sauce, 60, 94
Househ & Eggs, 108
hunter-gatherer, 45

I
immune system, 51, 57
inflammation, 18, 35, 51, 57, 60
inflammatory bowel, 15
ingredients, 67, 91
insulin, 58
intestinal wall, 29, 31, 35, 51, 52
intolerances, 18

J
Jerky, Beef, 100
Johnson, Barry, 99, 124
joint pain, 60
Joulwan, Melissa, 137
juice, 24, 25, 32, 34, 38, 57

K
kale, 32
Kayne, Jenni, 99, 130
kefir, 32
King Corn, 35
kombucha, 24, 32, 61
Kresser, Chris, 137

L
lactose, 32
Landy, Ray, 99, 120
lard, 25, 34
leaky gut, 35, 50, 51
lectins, 29, 32, 34, 35, 38, 51, 52, 55
legume(s), 24, 25, 29, 32, 33, 35, 38, 41, 45, 46, 52
lentils, 35
Lesage, Vincent, 99, 103
libido, 67
lifestyle, 63-71, 78
liver, 26, 60
Lott, Ronnie, 99, 122

ABOUT THE AUTHORS

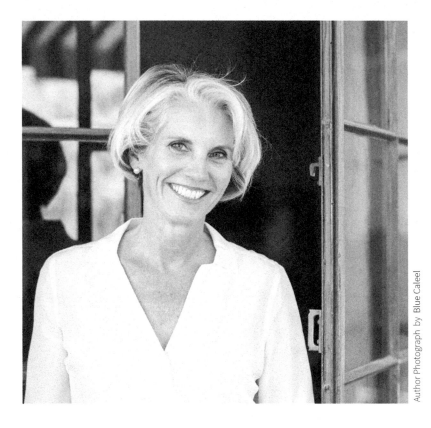

Author Photograph by Blue Caleel

CYNTHIA SPIVEY

Cynthia Spivey travels, eats and talks to people who will listen about her adventures with Paleo. She graduated from the University of California, Santa Barbara, with a degree in Communications & Media, which proved useful during her corporate writing career in New York City in the 1980s. She altered her career path to raise three children—born from her own womb in three different countries—while learning about cooking, nutrition and cultural foods. Based in Santa Barbara, California, her favorite Paleo treat is wine.

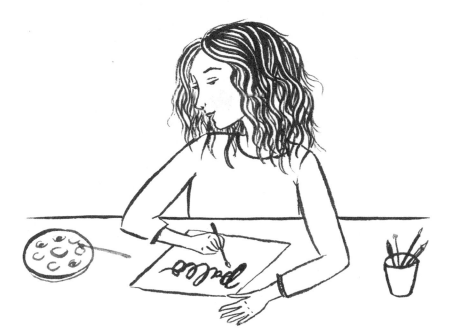

JOYA ROSE GROVES

Joya is a lettering artist and illustrator, happily painting and living with her husband in their seaside home of Carpinteria, California. After college Joya spent nearly two years abroad, journaling and illustrating her travels, which eventually led to embracing art as a career. This is her first illustrated book. Her favorite things are textured paper, her husband's cooking, mountaintops, picnics and a hot cup of tea on a cloudy day. Eggs from her parents' chickens are her favorite Paleo food.